DEMYSTIFYING
THE FEMALE BRAIN

A neuroscientist explores
health, hormones and happiness

DR SARAH MCKAY

First published in Great Britain in 2018 by Orion Spring
an imprint of The Orion Publishing Group Ltd
Carmelite House, 50 Victoria Embankment
London EC4Y 0DZ
An Hachette UK Company

1 3 5 7 9 10 8 6 4 2

A CIP catalogue record for this book is
available from the British Library.

ISBN: 978 1 4091 7318 2
Ebook ISBN: 978 1 4091 7319 9

Typeset in Garamond Regular by Kirby Jones
Printed in Great Britain by CPI Group (UK) Ltd, Croydon, CR0 4YY

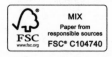

MIX
Paper from
responsible sources
FSC® C104740

www.orionbooks.co.uk

Every effort has been made to ensure that the information in the
book is accurate. The information in this book may not be applicable
in each individual case so it is advised that professional medical advice is
obtained for specific health matters and before changing any medication or dosage.
Neither the publisher nor author accepts any legal responsibility for any personal
injury or other damage or loss arising from the use of the information in this book.
In addition if you are concerned about your diet or exercise regime and wish
to change them, you should consult a health practitioner first.

DEMYSTIFYING
THE FEMALE BRAIN

Contents

Introduction

On being the owner and operator of a woman's brain

'Can you write an article on why women feel like they're losing their minds during menopause?' asked the editor of a brain health website I was writing for a few years ago. 'You're our neuroscience writer, see what you can find out.' My brief was straightforward: Write about the menopausal symptom 'brain fog' and its causes. When I set out to answer the question I rather naively assumed the answer would be simple – slow and hazy thinking, difficulty focusing, and forgetfulness (the more formal definitions of 'brain fog') could be blamed on ageing ovaries and waning hormones.

Digging into the research and speaking to women's health experts, I learned that it wasn't as simple as blaming brain fog on declining ovarian hormones. Levels of many hormones certainly do change with age and hormones impact how the brain works. However, each woman's individual experience of menopausal brain-related symptoms depends on multiple interacting causes such as her general level of health and wellbeing, genetic makeup, previous experience of depression, how much sleep or exercise she's getting, relationships and support networks, reproductive history and other life events.

I also discovered 'brain fog' differs from what doctors call mild cognitive impairment (MCI), which is a symptom of *unhealthy* brain ageing. Similarities between brain fog and MCI can cause considerable angst as many women mistakenly assume their fogginess indicates the beginning of the descent towards Alzheimer's disease (AD).

My wander into the world of women's brain health got me thinking about so-called 'baby brain', a term rather like 'brain fog' that some of my friends use to describe pregnancy-induced fuzzy thinking and an inability to concentrate. What are the causes of 'baby brain', I wondered? Could we lay the blame solely on pregnancy hormones? Was it due to anxiety around giving birth? Or was a kicking baby merely a distraction?

My musings over 'baby brain' and 'brain fog' and their causes triggered a cascade of questions about womanhood, nature, nurture and neurobiology that I'd never before considered.

Was postnatal depression due to plummeting hormones after giving birth, lack of sleep, or loss of identity as a career woman?

What about puberty blues? Was the emotional turmoil of adolescence due to the menstrual cycle? Or starting high school? Or mean girls?

What happens to our brains during the menstrual cycle? What impact does the pill have on our emotions? Is hormone replacement therapy (HRT) good or bad? Does motherhood change our brains? What happens to our brains when we fall in love?

I realised I'd spent forty-odd years as the owner and operator of a woman's body and brain, and over half of those years working as a neuroscientist, but I'd given close to zero consideration to how my neurobiology was sculpted by my life as a girl and woman, and indeed how my female brain influenced my everyday life and experiences.

And so, the idea for this book was born.

My goal is to take you on a chronological tour across the lifespan to explore how our minds and brains are shaped and sculpted by our genes and hormones, our life experiences, society and culture, and our thoughts, feelings and beliefs. The story begins in the womb and chapters focus in turn on infancy and girlhood, puberty and the menstrual cycle, the teenage years, mental health, romance and sex, pregnancy and motherhood, menopause, and finally longevity and old age. My focus is unashamedly on the female lifespan, but naturally, many of the themes explored apply equally to males and females, including in utero life, child and adolescent development, mental health, love and ageing.

Where is all the women's health neuroscience research?

Over the last decade writing about brain science, I've developed a tried and tested method for researching an unfamiliar topic. First, I'll read the appropriate chapter in *Principles of Neural Science*, the neuro-bible beloved by brain geeks the world over. Then I'll run a quick search on PubMed, an online search engine of biomedical literature, to find a recent review of the topic, typically written by a top scientist in the particular field, which will give me a feel for the topic's controversies and consensus. Then I'll feel confident enough to read and understand original research papers. Finally, I'll seek out the experts themselves – the scientists, doctors and specialists who, despite their busy schedules, usually give generously of their time to answer my questions and fill in the gaps of my knowledge.

However, describing the neurobiology of women's everyday lives hasn't always been as straightforward as I expected when I began. My meander through the world of women's health often left me bewildered. Time and time again I'd open the textbooks or scan the literature to find scant research on some of the questions I'd been most curious about.

For example, I assumed the literature would be replete with information on how the oral contraceptive pill affects women's brains. A 2014 review summed up the current state of affairs with the title *50 Years of Hormonal Contraception: Time to Find Out What It Does to the Brain*. Quite.

I proudly announced to Facebook the day I finally dived into the neurobiology of multiple orgasms. But it was not a deep dive. PubMed spat out only five literature reviews, three of which were devoted to the possibility of multiple orgasms in men. One was amusingly titled *Multiple Orgasms in Men: What We Know So Far*. (FYI: Orgasms don't rate a mention in neuroscience textbooks and we don't know much so far about women's orgasms either.)

Despite my best efforts, I was unable to pin down the statistics for how many women suffer emotional turmoil in the days leading up to their period, aka premenstrual syndrome (PMS). I eventually narrowed the range down to somewhere between twelve per cent and ninety per cent.

I was positive I'd be able to tell my mid-life readers whether or not HRT would help protect against dementia or clear away their brain fog. We simply don't have enough information about the benefits to brain health for any recommendations to be made. Why is the HRT literature so sparse when it comes to neurobiology and women's health?

There are a number of reasons.

Historically, preclinical research (research conducted on lab animals such as rats, mice or monkeys) has mostly been conducted on male animals. A 2009 survey of over 2000 animal studies found a significant male bias in eight out of ten biological disciplines. The bias was most pronounced in the field of neuroscience, where five and a half males were studied for every one female. Worryingly, pharmacology (the study of drugs) shares similar statistics, with five males studied to every one female.[1]

Clinical research (investigations conducted on humans) hasn't fared much better. There are a few large, all-female projects such as the Women's Health Study which I'll discuss in later chapters, but for many years women were excluded from clinical studies and drug trials altogether. As one critic notes, 'Many medical professionals can attest to the fact that for decades, the default human model subject was a 70-kg male.'[2]

This is alarming, because diagnoses for anxiety and depression are more than twice as common in women than in men, women have more strokes than men, twice as many women suffer from multiple sclerosis, and women have a higher susceptibility to adverse drug reactions compared with men. Indeed, between 1997 and 2000, eight out of ten drugs withdrawn from the US market were removed due to more severe adverse effects in women. The cumulative effect of excluding women from research studies, or assuming that biologically women are 'little men', is destructive.[3, 4] As has been pointed out in the journal *Nature*, medical care as it is currently applied to women is less evidence-based or 'robust' than that applied to men.[1]

You'd be tempted to believe that straightforward sexism permeates the hallowed halls and ivory towers as readily as other global institutions. It does, but sexism isn't the only reason for lack of gender equality. There are some legitimate reasons to skew the ratios. One reason is safety, because if women fall pregnant during a drug trial there is the potential for harming the unborn baby. Another reason is that females – both animals and humans – complicate data gathering. Our cyclical reproductive hormones, especially during the fertile years between puberty and menopause, make our biology intrinsically more fickle than males. The menstrual cycle was once likened to 'a pesky sort of feature essentially of the female, an unnecessary source of additional variability and one wisest to avoid'.[5]

To further complicate matters, in humans biological sex (anatomy and physiology) and gender (characteristics that a society or culture defines as masculine or feminine) are tightly entwined and hard to tease apart. As you'll learn, it's extraordinarily difficult to make statements such as, 'It's due to her hormones', or 'It's all to do with cultural expectations.' Rather than tackle the intricacies of female sex and gender, female hormones and culture, researchers often choose the easier route of focusing on males.

Finally, research on sex and gender was for a long time almost taboo. This was especially so in the neurosciences where many researchers were deeply concerned that their findings could be hijacked to support outdated and inaccurate stereotypes and discrimination. The fears were not unfounded. Women's brains have historically been found wanting or biologically inferior compared to men's, and such research has been co-opted to 'keep women in their place'.[6] One neuroscientist pointed out that exploring sex differences was once 'a terrific way for a brain scientist not studying reproductive functions to lose credibility at best and, at worst, become a pariah in the eyes of the neuroscience mainstream'.[5] I spoke to another who said she once believed including sex as a biological variable was 'lazy'. This was before she came to the conclusion that studying the impact of a woman's menstrual cycle on the brain might add a valuable dimension to her research.

Fortunately, the research community is taking steps to address the dearth of neurobiological research in women, and in this book you'll meet some of the researchers at the forefront of the movement. Institutions such as the National Institutes of Health (NIH) in the United States and academic publications such as the *Journal of Neuroscience Research* now mandate the inclusion of sex as a biological variable in all research. The World Health Organization (WHO) clearly states that research into health of women and girls is a particular priority. Here in Australia, we have the Australian Longitudinal Study on Women's Health, a survey of the physical, mental and psychosocial health of over 58 000 women across their lifespan. Finally, there are some fabulous research initiatives such as Stanford University's Gendered Innovations project that exist to 'harness the creative power of sex and gender analysis for innovation and discovery'.

How different are the differences between male and female brains?

Tell people you're writing a book about the neurobiology of women's everyday lives and you're inevitably asked the question, 'What are the differences between male and female brains?'

People are quick to rattle off a long list of attributes they believe are due to innate biological differences in the brains of men and women. We love the idea that all women have 'female brains', and all men possess 'male brains', and that in turn our brains govern our 'feminine' or 'masculine' behaviours, aptitudes, preferences and personality. You'll be familiar with some of these ideas.

Because of their 'female brains' women are emotional, can't read maps but can multitask, prefer people to things, don't ask for promotions, and certainly aren't cut out for computer coding or STEM careers.

Because of their 'male brains' men can't read emotions, prefer things to people (except when it comes to porn), are more likely to be geniuses, and aggressively seek higher status in the workplace.

Clearly, we're captivated by findings of sex and gender differences, especially when they're accompanied by a brain-based explanation. (Really, what could make a more seductive newspaper headline than a combination of sex and neuroscience?)

My answer to the sex difference question always begins with me stating that *this is not a book about the differences between male and female brains.* This book unashamedly explores girls' and women's health through the lens of neurobiology.

I then like to explain that there is no such thing as a 'male brain' or a 'female brain'. In fact, male and female brains are much more similar than they are different. We simply cannot sort people into two distinct groups based on their brain anatomy in the same way we can sensibly sort people into two groups based on the anatomy of their genitals. Instead, each of our brains are unique mosaics of different features, some male-like, some female-like, with plenty of features best described as androgynous.

The concept of a mosaic brain has received support from a group working at Tel Aviv University in Israel led by neurobiologist Daphna Joel. Her team used a type of brain-scanning technique called magnetic resonance imaging (MRI) to make hundreds of measurements of the brains of over 1400 adults. Joel's team found there was extensive overlap of the distributions of women and men for all brain regions and connections measured. Some brain features were more common in females compared with males, some more common in males compared with females, and up to half of the 1400 brains contained features common in both.[7]

Forgive the stereotypical colour selection, but think of it like this: our brains are assembled of many hundreds of little parts that are coloured pink if they are female-like and blue if they are male-like. Viewed from a distance, some women have brain mosaics that are strongly pink-tinged, others in men appear to be the bluest of blues, but most of us have brain mosaics coloured various shades of indigo, purple and mauve.

Another way to think about our brains is rather similarly to how we think about many of our habits, likes and dislikes, abilities and personality quirks: a mix of so-called 'masculine' or 'feminine' and gender-neutral characteristics. Each one of us is a unique mosaic and so is our brain.

There is a neat statistic that enables us to clearly assess the size of any sex difference. Now I'm very aware that for many of you, statistics may be dry and hard to conceptualise. Luckily neurobiologist Donna Maney has developed a nifty online tool you can use to give a clear illustration of the data. If you're so inclined, you can find it at SexDifference.org.

For the statistically minded, the tool generates a d value, which is a measure of the size of the difference between two groups. Here is the important part: if there is no sex difference, the d value is zero. As the size of the sex difference increases, the d value gets bigger. As a rule, a d value of up to 0.20 is considered a small sex difference, 0.50 is a moderate difference, and over 0.80 is a large difference.

Let's consider three examples of sex differences so you get the idea: adult height, connectivity between the left and right hemispheres of the brain, and maths scores at Year 3.

If I told you one of my parents was 191 centimetres tall and the other was 160 centimetres tall, you'd correctly guess the taller was my dad. There's no argument that the *average* man is taller than the *average* woman. However, we all know some women are taller than some men. So, if I told you I had a sibling who was 183 centimetres tall, you might guess I had a brother, when in fact I have a very tall sister. The large sex difference in average heights is reflected in a big *d* value of 1.91. Even so, there is still considerable overlap (about thirty-four per cent) between height distributions of men and women.

One popular claim is that women's left and right hemispheres are 'more connected' than men's hemispheres because we have a bigger corpus callosum (the fibre bundle that bridges the two sides of the brain). For some reason, this has been taken to mean women excel at multitasking and expressing empathy. In Figure 1, you'll see there is a difference in the average connectivity between males and females, but it's small. The *d* value is 0.31 with eighty-eight per cent overlap.

Another notion is that boys are better at maths than girls (apparently this explains why there aren't many female software engineers working for Google). To test this claim I put the scores from the 2016 Year 3 NAPLAN numeracy test (an Australia-wide standardised test[8]), which is the year my oldest son completed the exams, into Maney's SexDifference.org calculator. For my son's cohort, the boys' average maths score was ever so slightly higher than the girls' average score. But the *d* value was 0.14, meaning the difference was trivial, and the overlap between distributions was ninety-four per cent. In other words, nearly half the girls scored higher marks than the average boy.

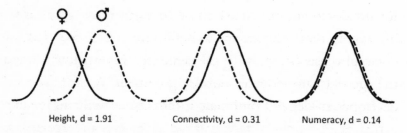

Figure 1. Distribution curves for sex differences in adult height, left-right brain hemisphere connectivity and numeracy. Solid line = females. Dashed line = males. Adapted from sexdifference.org

The idea behind these statistics is not to bore you to tears but to give you a practical way to assess reported sex differences using a valid scientific tool. If you so wish to spend your time, any decent scientific report should contain all the data you need to plug into the calculator.

By introducing the concept of mosaic brains and the statistics of sex differences versus similarities, I'm not trying to minimise or sidestep discussions of any differences that do exist. Rather, I'd like to encourage you out of the habit of asking 'Are we different?' and instead ask more sophisticated questions such as, 'What is the size of the difference? What are the similarities? What is my individual brain like?'

Clearly, the extent and nature of physical, psychological and behavioural differences in the brains of human females and males is highly controversial and politicised. Professor Margaret McCarthy, a neuroscientist who studies sex hormones and the developing brain, tactfully sums up the controversy by stating, 'Sex differences in the brain are more than some would like and less than others believe.'[9]

Nature, nurture or neuroplasticity?

I've always been intrigued by how our brains are shaped by our lives, and how in turn our brains shape who we are. So, for my doctorate research I chose to explore the very earliest life events that influence how brain circuitry is sculpted. My doctoral thesis begins with the sentence, 'My work will revisit the age-old nature versus nurture argument. What features of development depend on innate mechanisms, and what require experience?'

For three years I ran overnight experiments in a dusty ground-floor corner room in the University Laboratory of Physiology at

Oxford. I painstakingly documented the development of brain cells (neurons) and their connections (synapses) in the visual cortex (the part of the brain that processes vision). I hoped to define which aspects of brain circuitry were shaped by innate biological mechanisms (nature) and which depended on life experiences (nurture).

The final page of my thesis concludes, 'In summary, it appears the circuitry of the brain changes during development. Both nature and nurture are involved.' And when asked the inevitable question, 'How's the thesis?' by my graduate friends over pints in a pub, all I could offer for my years of sleep deprivation was, 'I found out the brain changes. It's not nature *or* nurture. I think it's probably a bit of both.'

My research didn't add anything too unexpected to the field but the results were neatly in line with the extensive body of literature supporting the view nature *and* nurture are necessary for wiring up brain circuits during development.

That was twenty years ago, and today there's no longer a philosophical debate about which matters more. Nature and nurture cooperate. They work in synergy. Our brain is sculpted by genes, hormones, molecules and the innate patterns of neural activity that make up the 'nature' program, and by our childhood experiences, social connections, education, culture, and the world around us, all of which make up the 'nurture' program. Together, nature and nurture sculpt a brain.

Your plastic mosaic brain

Closely related to the notion that the brains of men and women are different is the idea that any differences are permanently hardwired by genes or hormone exposure in the womb. The assumption is that nature matters, nurture doesn't. The belief that the brains of men and women are intrinsically different completely overlooks the fact that sex and gender, like nature and nurture, interact.

The misconception that sex differences are innate and therefore fixed flies in the face of the well-established fact that our brains are plastic and continue to change our whole lives. In one sense, brain development is never really 'finished' until we die. Every experience we have – from reading the words of this book, to entering puberty, to interacting with co-workers, to running a race, to loving a child – shapes our brains. The trillions of connections are continually flourishing or being pruned back, forming and re-forming, moulding and refining to fit our environment.

The pink and blue pieces of the brain mosaic are not hardened fragments of ceramic glued in place in the womb, guided to their final positions by genes and prenatal hormones. Instead, pieces are removed, remoulded, replaced, polished and honed throughout our lives. Our mosaic brains are plastic and distinctive artworks in progress.

Because the aim of this book is not to spend time exploring the science of sex differences (and similarities), nor to smash apart Mars versus Venus gender stereotypes, I recommend interested readers check out two excellent books: *Delusions of Gender: The Real Science Behind Sex Differences* by feminist psychologist Cordelia Fine,[10] and *Pink Brain, Blue Brain: How Small Differences Grow into Troublesome Gaps – and What We Can Do About It* by neuroscientist Lise Eliot.[11]

A disclaimer

As a neuroscientist I was schooled not only in physiology, pharmacology and psychology, but also how to assess the weight of evidence, consider various hypotheses and generate alternative explanations based on data. Academic papers also come with a series of disclaimers, outlining caveats of the work.

Here are mine, to keep in mind when reading this book:

Sex is biological and usually, but not always, straightforward. For some people, gender and sex are not as simple as 'XX chromosomes make a girl' and 'XY chromosomes make a boy'. We're now learning more about infants born with intersex conditions where their reproductive or sexual anatomy don't fit the typical definitions of female or male.

Gender is much more complicated again. Gender is a combination of cultural, social, biological and psychological elements. Gender is how we look, act and feel. More often than not, gender and sex are aligned. In this case, a baby born with female genitals and presumably two X chromosomes grows up identifying as a girl or woman. Similarly, a baby born with a penis and presumably male XY chromosomes grows up identifying as a boy or man. People for whom gender identity and biological sex are in alignment are often referred to as 'cisgender'. The terminology for people whose gender and sex don't match varies, but includes terms such as transgender, non-binary and gender non-conforming.[12]

Sexual orientation is different again and includes feelings of attraction (emotional, psychological, physical and/or sexual) towards other people. A person may be attracted to people of the same sex, to those of the opposite sex, to those of both sexes, or without reference to sex or gender at all.[12]

Unless I state otherwise, when I use terms like 'girl' or 'woman' in this book, I'm referring to people who were born with female genitals, presumably with two X chromosomes; who were raised as girls and now identify as women. I'm very aware there are many people who don't fit this traditional classification, and including discussions of the neurobiology of intersex, transgendered or transsexual people would clearly enrich a book such as this; however, as there is often scant neuroscience research available, mostly this book is about cisgender girls and women.

Determination of sex and gender are complex and the science is only just catching up on the reality of the spectrum. For those readers curious to learn more about the science 'beyond' the textbook definitions of male and female, sex and gender, the September 2017 issue of *Scientific American*, 'Sex and Gender: It's Not a Women's Issue', provides a wonderfully useful overview.[13]

You'll see I share some of my own stories in this book. I'm a cisgender straight woman, but I'm in no way implying my experiences represent the experiences of other women.

1.

In Utero

The Great Sperm Race

Armed with graph paper, a thermometer and a textbook understanding of the hormonal control of ovulation, I approached the business of trying to conceive with the earnest enthusiasm of a first-year PhD student. Fortunately, my body and husband cooperated and I've been a mum to two beautiful boys for the best part of a decade. While writing this chapter it came time for my husband to take our eldest son to the requisite 'Where did I come from?' evening at school. I waited impatiently at home and when they arrived back (and despite my best attempt at cool, nonchalant parenting), my son had barely walked in the door when I asked, 'So, where DO babies come from?'

'Well, it's weird, embarrassing, but interesting too,' he said. 'The sperms swim up the channel. Half go the wrong way and die. The other half go the right way and find the egg, which is releasing a chemical. One sperm locks in and is the winner.'

The moment the winning sperm 'locks in' to the egg and bequeaths either an X or Y chromosome is life defining, and weird but interesting too. For most people, if you're a biological female, you inherited one X chromosome from your mother and one X from your father. If you are biologically a male, you inherited your X chromosome from your mother and the Y from your father.

The two sex chromosomes get their names because they look like the letters 'X' and 'Y' under a microscope. Along with another twenty-two pairs, chromosomes consist of two tightly wound double strands of DNA. DNA contains the instructions for our genes, and genes are the instructions for making proteins. Our complete DNA instruction manual contains surprisingly few genes – about 20000 – of which one-third contain the instructions for building the brain.[14]

The average neuron makes tens of thousands of connections, called synapses, with other neurons. And even if we're conservative, a brain of 86 billion neurons may contain as many as one hundred trillion synapses. If you're savvy, you'll realise that the maths don't add up: we have too many synapses for too few genes.

It turns out the relationships between our genes, brains and behaviour are utterly complex. The DNA we inherited from our mother and father influences who we are, but not in a direct and simple way. In this book, we'll explore how those trillions of synapses in the female brain make us who we are. You'll see that while genes provide the basic biological instructions for life, many other biological, social and psychological elements interact, synergise and alter the expression of genes.

Implanting the egg

Strictly speaking, the fertilised egg is called a zygote. For its first six to seven days of life the zygote bumps and rolls down the fallopian tube dividing multiple times until it becomes a hollow ball of cells, called a blastocyst. Once the blastocyst reaches the uterus it embeds in the uterine wall, where cells keep dividing until the ball organises into two layers: one layer becomes the embryo and the other becomes the placenta.[15]

The placenta is not merely an interface between a baby and her mother. It acts as a giant gland releasing an assortment of hormones and chemical messengers crucial for maintaining pregnancy and preparing mum-to-be for birth. The placenta's first job is to manufacture the pregnancy hormone human Chorionic Gonadotropin (hCG). If you've ever anxiously waited for a thin blue line to appear after peeing on a pregnancy test, it's an hCG chemical reaction you're waiting for. hCG also triggers the cascade of hormones that stop your menstrual cycle.[16]

Because the placenta derives from the same cells as the baby-to-be, either XX or XY, it too has a biological sex. Placental sex determines how the placenta works and how it buffers the baby against maternal stress, infection and diet. The placenta is central to sex differences in prenatal growth and survival, and the female placenta appears to be somewhat protective compared to the male.[17]

The case of the neural tube is not yet closed

By the time your pregnancy test is positive, or you skip a period (roughly two weeks after conception, or four weeks from your last period), your baby's brain has begun to form. The nervous system is one of the earliest body systems to begin development and is one of the last to finish – our brains continue to mature well into our twenties and thirties.

The human brain and spinal cord arise from the neural plate, which is a flattened layer of cells in the embedded blastocyst. Following a well-orchestrated sequence of steps the flattened layer of cells folds, the edges bend to touch in the middle, close over and 'zipper up' to form a neural tube. Concerning ourselves with early events in brain development might seem overly detail-focused, but this phase is momentous because the entire nervous system emerges from the neural tube.

You may have heard the term 'neural tube' spoken of before, usually in a very serious tone alongside the phrases 'take your folic acid supplements' and 'birth defect'. Rightly so. The intricate and complex process of neural tube closure can go very wrong, and folate appears to play a protective role. Folate is the naturally occurring form of Vitamin B9 and is called folic acid when manufactured.

If the neural tube fails to close correctly by twenty-eight days after conception a number of serious birth abnormalities can result, including spina bifida and anencephaly (literally meaning absence of brain). For all the evidence that folate prevents neural tube defects, the exact mechanisms by which the essential vitamin contributes to the zippering up of the neural tube is still a mystery. As some researchers have quipped, the case of folate and the neural tube is far from closed.[18]

You were destined to be female

You might be wondering when I'll address *female* brain development. The main reason I've been using androgynous terms so far is because for the first month or so after conception, male and female embryos are indistinguishable. Bear with me, because to understand female brain development we must first discuss male embryonic development.

When XY embryos are six to eight weeks old, a gene on the Y chromosome called the 'sex-determining region of the Y chromosome', or SRY for short, turns on. SRY contains the instructions for building a protein called 'testis determining factor', which guides development of the testes. SRY kickstarts a cascade of dozens of genes that are turned on in male embryos and turned off in female embryos.[19]

Jenny Graves, a professor of genetics at La Trobe University, explains that even though SRY is just one gene, the downstream effects of SRY are much more profound than simply building testicles. 'Male hormones, such as testosterone, are synthesised by the embryonic testis and have far-flung effects all over the developing body. Androgens turn on hundreds (maybe thousands) of genes that determine male genitalia, male growth, hair, voice and elements of behaviour,' she says.[20]

In the *absence* of a Y chromosome the default developmental option is for the foetus to become a female.

'Default' is a term some people find a little dismissive.

To help unravel the complexities of male versus female prenatal brain development, I called Margaret McCarthy, a professor of neuroscience who studies the effects of hormones on brain development at the University of Maryland School of Medicine. McCarthy is one of the pioneers in the field and conducted some of the first studies on how sex hormones organise the developing brain. 'Default does not mean passive,' was one of the first things she said to me in a tone of voice that had me convinced she's made that statement more than once. 'Try using "the developing mammalian brain is *destined* for a female phenotype," instead,' she suggested.

So now we know, all embryos are *destined* to become female, unless the SRY gene in the Y chromosome turns on.

Ovaries develop in the absence of the Y male chromosome

An XX foetus has no Y chromosome, therefore no SRY gene; instead, other genes are turned on and off to actively promote the ovarian development program and suppress the testes program.

Ovaries are just one in a trio of structures that coordinate much of our reproductive lives. The trio goes by the name 'Hypothalamic-Pituitary-Ovarian axis' (HPO axis) and consists of ovaries, and two brain structures called the hypothalamus and pituitary gland.

Let's take a brief look at the trio of structures, starting with the hypothalamus. It is found at the base of your brain under the thalamus (hence the name 'hypo-thalamus') next to its partner, the pituitary gland. Of all the regions of the brain, the hypothalamus is one of the busiest. It monitors and maintains the life essentials of temperature control, metabolism, hunger, thirst, aggression, sexual arousal, circadian rhythms and stress. It's elaborately connected to other brain regions via neural pathways, and to the rest of the body by its rich supply of blood vessels, thus enabling it to coordinate the brain's response to the body.

The close proximity of the hypothalamus and the pituitary gland is important, as hormones and other neurochemicals from the hypothalamus are secreted into a series of blood vessels that connect directly to the anterior pituitary. This portal allows for rapid and direct communication.

The anterior pituitary is often referred to as the 'master gland' because its hormones stimulate and coordinate glands, tissue and organs elsewhere, including the ovaries. But the term master gland is a misnomer, because the pituitary's master is the hypothalamus, which tightly controls all action that takes place.

Finally, we have the ovaries. They're found tucked away in the lower abdomen, far, far away from the brain. Ovaries produce and release hormones and eggs (oocytes), and by halfway through her time in utero, a baby girl's ovaries contain about five million oocytes. In a developmental theme that will shortly become familiar to you, two-thirds of these oocytes die off such that a newborn has about half to one million oocytes. By the time she reaches puberty, a girl's oocyte count will have dwindled to a few hundred thousand. Give or take a few pregnancies, on average 450 eggs will be released over the course of her lifetime.

Ovaries respond to hormonal signals from the pituitary that arrive via the bloodstream by secreting hormones of their own – primarily oestrogen during the first half of the menstrual cycle, but also the hormone progesterone once ovulation is established. As they mature, they get better at responding to signals from the brain, and part of this maturation is reflected in the 'settling' of the menstrual cycle during early adolescence. It can take a few years for a mature ovulation cycle to be established.

From puberty, one of the most important roles of the HPO axis is to regulate release of ovarian hormones including oestrogen. Oestrogen isn't a single hormone; rather *oestrogens* are a group of three hormones: oestradiol, oestriol and oestrone.

♀ *Oestradiol* is the main oestrogen manufactured by the ovaries. It is important for the development of secondary sex characteristics such as breasts, and for the menstrual cycle and pregnancy. Synthetic versions of oestradiol are used in contraceptive pills.

♀ *Oestriol* is made by the placenta. Oestriol is barely detectable unless you're pregnant, when levels increase 1000-fold.

♀ *Oestrone* is another less-potent oestrogen produced by the ovaries and it doesn't dominate till after menopause.

To keep things simple, and unless it's important to differentiate between the three oestrogens, I'll use the umbrella term 'oestrogen' throughout this book.

Sex hormones organise reproductive regions of the prenatal brain

Mother Nature is selfish. Her one and only goal is for us to have sex and make babies. To ensure dating and mating occurs, the parts of our brain that control reproduction, in particular the hypothalamus, become 'masculinised' or 'feminised' to match our male or female gonads.

Hormones influence how these reproductive brain circuits grow and respond. Prenatal life is the first of two life phases when the brain is super-sensitive to sex hormones. 'We call this early period of hormone exposure the organisational period, as it organises or programs the brain to respond to hormones in adulthood,' explains McCarthy. Many sex differences that do exist are developmentally organised and then activated, or revealed, by the action of hormones during the second phase, puberty.

During the prenatal period, the dominating influence is that of testosterone produced by foetal testes. Testosterone helps to ensure that the reproductive regions of the brain in males become masculinised. At the same time, and in the *absence* of testosterone, brain regions involved in reproductive behaviours in females become feminised.

What is the role of oestrogen in female brain development?

You might be wondering, if testosterone 'masculinises' the unborn baby boy, does oestrogen from foetal ovaries play a role in in 'feminising' the unborn baby girl?

Believe it or not, foetal oestrogen plays no role at all. Female embryos do not require ovarian hormones to become feminised (remember, they're *destined* to become female). Oestrogen's role in the developing female brain is thus a by-product of its *absence*, rather than presence.

Unborn babies' brains are also shielded from the influence of maternal oestrogens (made by their mother and the placenta) by a molecule called alpha-fetoprotein, which is made in the liver of an unborn baby. It binds to oestrogen in the bloodstream and prevents maternal oestrogen crossing into the baby's brain.[21]

Curiously, oestrogen is involved in organising the architecture of the *male* brain. Testosterone easily passes into unborn baby boys' brains where it is converted to oestradiol by an enzyme called aromatase. It is now well established that the 'female' hormone oestradiol is responsible for 'masculinising' the male brain in utero.

Mother Nature is selfish. And she also has a sense of humour.

Joining the dots from brain to behaviour

Sex differences in achievement in maths, interest in technology subjects or ability in the sciences are often solely attributed to the presence (or absence) of testosterone in the womb. In 2005, Harvard University president Lawrence Summers controversially suggested that innate biological differences (namely, prenatal testosterone) explain why men have more career success in mathematics than women – he later resigned.

A Google software engineer trotted out the same argument in August 2017 to explain why fewer women succeed in STEM careers than men and to rail against diversity training – he was fired.

Most scientists who study sex differences agree the weight of evidence finds prenatal testosterone doesn't directly determine adult academic achievement or career choice. Cordelia Fine points out that investigations of sex differences due to hormones are often correlational, and they tend to imply that hormonal level is the primary cause, rather than taking into account the fact that our biology is 'entangled' with our life experiences and social context.[22]

Prenatal hormones may provide 'a small push in one direction'.[11] That early 'push' can be either enhanced or entirely eliminated by how girls and boys are raised. My thinking is this: it was rare for women to work as politicians, lawyers and doctors even sixty years ago. There were few female scientists, engineers or mathematicians (and possibly very few women authoring neuroscience books). It's clear to me that small sex differences apparent in the brains of unborn infants cannot reliably explain the enormous gender inequalities we see in society. Our society's attitudes and cultural expectations of the capabilities of girls and women and our place in the workplace have changed dramatically. Prenatal hormone levels haven't.

It's proving much harder than you might think for neuroscientists to draw a straight line from prenatal hormones to brain to behaviour. We struggle to connect the dots in carefully controlled studies of rodents in the research lab, let alone in humans. This can be attributed most simply to the fact that extensive *networks* of brain cells control who we are and how we behave. One role of those networks is to integrate multiple sources of information. Throughout the lifespan, social, cultural and psychological influences combine with biology in complex ways to determine how we think, feel and behave.

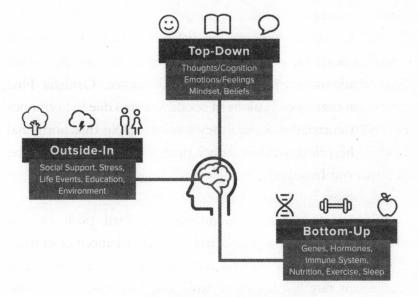

Figure 2. The Bottom-Up Outside-In Top-Down Model.

I developed the Bottom-Up Outside-In Top-Down model for my students to provide a framework within which to consider how biological, psychological and social factors impact on the brain over the lifespan.

♀ Bottom-Up elements are the biological or physiological determinants of brain health, development and ageing. They include genes, hormones, the immune system, nutrition, exercise, sleep and other lifestyle choices we make.

♀ Outside-In elements include your social circle, living environment, life events, education, current circumstances, external stressors and family background.

♀ Top-Down elements include thoughts, emotions, personality, mindset and belief systems.

Not only do these many elements regulate the development, performance and health of the brain, each element influences others in dynamic ways.

For example:

- ♀ Our thoughts and feelings can influence our physical experience of pain, which is why outside-in stress can exacerbate top-down perceptions of bottom-up pain.
- ♀ Social connection can directly impact our brain health, which is why folks who are socially isolated are at greater risk of dementia.
- ♀ Our physical health and mood are intimately entwined, which is why bottom-up exercise is key for top-down emotional regulation and can be used to treat depression.

How to build a brain

If you've ever attended a neurosurgery (or watched one on YouTube), you might have noticed that living human brains are neither pink nor blue. They're a pulsating purplish grey. The wrinkly outermost layer of cortex, the grey matter, gets its name from its appearance, and it contains cell bodies of neurons, their branching extensions called dendrites and other cell types called glia. A centimetre below the surface runs white matter consisting of nerve bundles that connect different regions of grey matter together.

Traditionally, the cortex is subdivided into four lobes per hemisphere: frontal, temporal, parietal and occipital. Broadly speaking, each lobe has a job: the occipital lobes process vision; the temporal lobes process sound, speech and memory; parietal lobes integrate our senses and movement; and the frontal lobes, which are larger and more evolved by far in humans than any other creature, control movement, language, abstract reasoning and attention.

How do we know which part of the brain does what? The opening line of Oliver Sacks's masterpiece *The Man Who Mistook His Wife for a Hat* gives us a clue: 'Neurology's favourite word is deficit.' Deficits in function caused by a stroke perhaps, or a brain tumour, gave neurologists their first insight into what is called 'localisation of function'.[23]

As Sacks tells us, the scientific study of the relationship between the brain and mind began in 1861 when French neurologist Paul Broca found speech problems always followed damage to a particular portion of the left temporal lobe. This opened the way to mapping the human brain, ascribing specific powers − linguistic, intellectual, emotional, visual and so on − to equally specific parts of the brain. During my PhD I spent hundreds of hours poking tungsten micro-electrodes four millimetres deep into the portion of occipital cortex where I knew with certainty I could record inputs from one eye or the other. Similarly, neurosurgeons use stimulating electrodes to carefully map the brain before they pick up their scalpel, thus avoiding damaging critical regions. Modern-day functional MRI (fMRI) maps blood flow as a stand-in for brain activity and therefore localisation of function.

A particular job or trait is never 'hardwired' into a specific cortical location for life. Remember, our brains are plastic and change in response to experience. During my tungsten micro-electrode recording sessions I was able to manipulate an individual neuron's preference for the left or right eye depending on whether one or the other eye was blindfolded. Other researchers have shown visual neurons can even learn to respond to sound if neural inputs from the ear are encouraged to reroute. This capacity for plasticity underlies our ability to learn and remember, and to recover from brain injury such as stroke.

Dig a little deeper and we see the brain's regional specificity is supported by diversity. Even the seemingly simplest of neural structures is made up of a huge assortment of cell types. In the retina of the eye there are dozens of classes of neuron, and in the spinal cord more than one hundred different types of specialised neurons project to muscles. Diversity comes about in the early embryo by way of chemical gradients and signalling molecules. Head-to-tail or left–right patterns, for example, are determined by how near or far a cell is from a source of a chemical that influences which genes switch on or off, thereby determining what type of cell develops.

The diversity and the precise connections formed by many billions of neurons during in utero development underlie the wondrous capacity of our brains and minds. A brain that allows us to love, feel, move through the world, create artworks, send satellites into space and even, when damaged as Sacks's patient's brain was, 'reach out his hand, take hold of his wife's head, try to lift it off and put it on'.

The birth of new brain cells

Going from a few hundred cells rolled up in a neural tube to the 86 billion extraordinarily diverse cell types present in a newborn's brain involves a colossal amplification of numbers. Simple maths tells us that a quarter to a half a million neurons are born per minute during in utero life. The proliferation of massive numbers of brain cells comes down to one type of cell – the stem cell.

Stem cells evoke images of crazy scientists, hopeful therapies for cancer and Parkinson's disease, and ethical controversies over using aborted human foetal tissue. But their natural existence is rather less melodramatic.

Stem cells possess a couple of unique qualities: they divide endlessly, making multiple copies of themselves, and they can differentiate into any cell type found in the body. *Neural* stem cells, as their name suggests, produce all cell types found in the brain and nervous system, including both neurons and glia. The process by which neurons are born from stem cells is called *neurogenesis*, and when glia are born the process is called *gliogenesis*.

Glia make up half the cells in the brain and come in three main subtypes: astrocytes, oligodendrocytes, and microglia. The word 'glia' is Greek for 'glue', because it was once assumed glia existed solely to 'glue' neurons in place. But glia provide much more than structural support. They offer nutritional support to neurons, clear toxins while we sleep (astrocytes), insulate the axons of neurons with myelin (oligodendrocytes, or Schwann cells in the peripheral nervous system), and act as the brain's innate immune system (microglia). Gliogenesis persists across the human lifespan and the losses and gains of oligodendrocytes, for example, can be visualised in brain scans as changes in volume or density of white matter.

Neurogenesis in the adult human brain is less well understood. Neurogenesis was first described in middle-aged people in a landmark paper using atmospheric Carbon-14 levels, a type of carbon atom generated by nuclear bombs that becomes integrated into DNA. From 1955 to 1963, there were elevated atmospheric Carbon-14 levels caused by above-ground nuclear bomb testing during the cold war. Carbon-14 reacts with oxygen to form CO_2, which is taken up by plants in photosynthesis, and when we eat plants, or animals that live off plants, we take up Carbon-14 into cells that are dividing creating a 'date mark' in the DNA. For people alive during the Cold War years, any newborn neurons in their brains became 'tagged' with Carbon-14. Using this innovative strategy, neuroscientists estimate 700 new Carbon-14-tagged neurons are born in each middle-aged human hippocampus daily. The hippocampus (from the Greek for 'seahorse', which it resembles) is the brain's centre for learning and memory.[24]

Understandably, there is plenty of excitement around neurogenesis, in particular its therapeutic prospects and implications for brain ageing. After all, who doesn't love the notion we continually add new brain cells daily rather than losing them as we age? While seemingly impressive, 700 neurons per day represents only 0.004 per cent of the total of one cell type in the hippocampus and that figure is ten-fold lower than seen in the rodents used to model neurological diseases. So some scientists question how such a relatively small number of newborn neurons contribute to complex behaviours and psychiatric disorders.[25] To dampen your enthusiasm a little further, you should realise that the vast majority of neurogenesis research has since been done in lab animals, not humans. We know rodent neurogenesis is slowed by stress, depression or inflammation, and sped up by antidepressants, exercise and learning. However, we simply don't know if the same happens in adult human brains.

Zika virus disrupts brain cell migration

In late 2015, global newspapers started reporting on the unusually large numbers of babies born with shrunken malformed heads (microcephaly) in South America, in particular Brazil. There were plenty of theories flying round, but most evidence pointed towards an outbreak of mosquito-born Zika virus as the cause. In the run-up to the 2016 Rio Olympics many international travellers and athletes considered skipping the games to avoid the threat.

It turns out Zika virus infects a type of brain cell called 'radial glia'.

Besides acting as neural stem cells, radial glia provide the scaffold along which newborn neurons migrate. If you were to slice a section through the developing neural tube you'd see radial glia spanning the thickness of the wall of the tube, rather like spokes in a bike wheel. Once neurons are born, they crawl from the inside of the tube along radial glia until they reach their home. Each subsequent newborn neuron crawls over the top of those already nestled into place, such that the six layers of cortex develop in an inside-first outside-last fashion. In this way, the birthdate of a neuron determines its final postcode. Once their crucial roles in development are complete, radial glia retract their processes, ball up and differentiate into astrocytes.

At the time of writing, research points towards Zika infection of radial glia being the cause of defects in babies whose mothers contracted the virus when pregnant. When the Zika virus infects radial glial cells, it stops their growth, division and survival, which in turn cuts the number of neurons born and migrating into position. This may be the mechanism by which babies are being born with grossly underdeveloped brains.[26, 27]

Half of all neurons are born to die

In a healthy pregnancy, the vast majority of neurogenesis is complete by about months five to six. Then something rather unexpected happens: half of all the neurons that have been born die.

Neurons die via a highly regulated process of cellular suicide called *apoptosis*; derived from the Greek word for leaves falling off a tree. It sounds wasteful, but apoptosis is important for establishing final numbers of neurons and glia, and for matching the number of neurons to the size of the final targets that they innervate. Outside of the brain, the role of apoptosis is clearer: a foetus's hand starts out as a flattened webbed-like structure similar to a duck's foot; to reveal human-like fingers, the cells in the webbed tissue between the fingers shrivel and die by apoptosis.

Molecules guide axons to their targets

'The brain is a world consisting of a number of unexplored continents and great stretches of unknown territory,' wrote Santiago Ramón y Cajal, a Spanish neuroscientist and 1906 Nobel laureate, often referred to as the godfather of modern neuroscience.

Cajal was right. After birth and migration to their final postcode, and if they're not the fifty per cent pre-programmed to die, all neurons sprout projections. Many of the projections, called dendrites, look rather like the branches of a tree and act as the neuron's input-receivers – they listen in to signals being sent to them from other neurons. The output structure of the neuron, the axon, is a long slender vine-like projection that transmits electrical signals away from the neuron's cell body. Once the neuron settles into its home and sprouts projections, the long vine-like axon sets off on a secondary migration all of its own.

The growing tip of the axon called the growth cone is a wonder. It's a sensory structure that can navigate by following the molecular and chemical signposts in the environment, and a motor whose activity physically propels the axon across the terrain of the foetal brain. Axons can project short distances and connect to neighbours mere microns away, or extend over metres (all the way down the spinal cord to your big toe) – a navigational feat likened to a baby crawling from Perth, say, to a Sydney harbourside apartment building and managing to knock on the correct door. Once the growing axon reaches its destination, the growth cone collapses and differentiates into a specialised structure called a synapse.

Synapses are miniature zones of communication

Two neurons don't touch; instead, they are separated by the smallest of gaps called a synapse. The purpose of a synapse is to convert an electrical signal into a chemical signal, which carries the message across the narrow synaptic cleft, where it's converted back into an electrical signal by the receiving neuron.

You will have heard of some of the most famous signalling chemicals, neurotransmitters such as dopamine, oxytocin, and serotonin. Despite their fame, neurons containing them are comparatively rare in the brain, and they merely modify the actions of the two major neurotransmitters: glutamate, which excites neural activity, and GABA, which inhibits neural activity. Changes in the structure and numbers of synapses are fundamental to how our brains change. Most psychoactive drugs, from coffee to nicotine to cocaine to antidepressants, act at the synapse. And as we'll learn in later chapters, synapses are modified by learning and experience. This is known as synaptic plasticity and endows each of us with our individual brains.

Use it or lose it

In early development, there is a massive superabundance of synapses. Far more connections are made than are required. So, rather like the fifty per cent of neurons that die, superfluous synapses are pruned away.

Prenatal synaptic pruning can go wrong, and when it does it can result in a rather intriguing condition called synaesthesia. As Oliver Sacks described, normally each area of our brain is specialised for the processing of information from one type of input. For people with synaesthesia, inappropriate pruning of synapses leaves the 'wrong' brain areas connected together. People with synaesthesia can 'hear' colours or 'taste' shapes, and their descriptions of how they perceive the world might include, 'January is a pale apple-green colour' or 'The note middle C tastes like beef stock.' Such rich, creative portrayals of the world are typical for about four per cent of the population who don't suffer so much as are *gifted* with synaesthesia.

The first 1000 days of brain development

There are roughly 1000 days from conception until a child reaches her second birthday. These first 1000 days have emerged as a critical window of opportunity in which to build the foundation for a child's ability to grow, learn, and contribute in the future.

What can we do to support the first 280 of the 1000 days?

As we know, adequate folate in the diet or via supplements reduces the risk of neural tube defects. Alcohol and smoking are also the other two obvious avoidable sources of harm. Babies of mothers who drink excessively during pregnancy show reduced brain growth and brain volume, and the microstructure of their neurons and synapses is altered. Nicotine affects axonal pathfinding and synapse formation, and carbon monoxide inhaled from cigarettes leads to foetal hypoxia (lack of oxygen), all of which thwart normal brain development.[28] Interestingly, boys are more likely to suffer the effects of maternal smoking than girls. This might be linked to the protective effects of the female placenta.[29]

Worrying about worry

During my first pregnancy it felt like so much could go wrong – imagine if I inhaled passive smoke or forgot my pregnancy vitamins? Years researching brain development made me way too aware of how sensitive the prenatal period is for baby humans. I found pregnancy very stressful. And when my mum reminded me that 'stressing out' was going to stress my baby I naturally started feeling stressed about how stressed I was feeling.

During a healthy pregnancy, levels of the stress hormone cortisol rise two to three fold but the baby is buffered from 'normal but high' maternal cortisol by an enzyme in the placenta. However, it's thought that extreme stress or trauma – such as that caused by natural disasters, violence or serious illness – can modify the activity of the enzyme, potentially 'transferring' the stress to the baby. Overexposure of cortisol in utero is thought to be one of the key mechanisms linking early life development with later life disease. What happens in the womb at different points in development can affect the baby after birth, during childhood and well into adulthood – a concept known as 'foetal programming'.[30]

For once, my mum was wrong. *Normal* levels of maternal angst don't harm unborn babies. In fact, angst might have the opposite effect. One study of ninety-four healthy women by Johns Hopkins University researchers found that 'non-clinical maternal anxiety' (i.e., the typical level of worrying by a first-time parent) or non-specific pregnancy stress (e.g. worrying how much the baby is moving) was *beneficial* to the babies. Children born to mothers who exhibited high versus low levels of non-clinical maternal anxiety and non-specific stress showed more advanced motor and cognitive development at age two.[31]

The authors say they hope their findings may provide relief to women who have a tendency to worry about worrying. I wish I'd known about this study when I was pregnant!

The Montreal Ice Storm Study

Natural disasters provide a convenient if unfortunate 'natural experiment' for looking at how very stressful events can impact brain development before birth. One such natural experiment took place in the Canadian province of Quebec in January 1998 when an ice storm dumped so much frozen rain on the city, thousands of transmission towers collapsed under the weight of ice. The electricity grid was crippled and three million people, including hundreds of pregnant women, were without power for at least forty-five days at the most brutally cold time of the year.

Five months after the disaster, a team from McGill University, led by psychiatrist Suzanne King, saw a unique opportunity. The ice storm would enable them to study the effects of maternal stress on the development of children who were in utero at the time. King's team recruited a few hundred women who had been pregnant during the disaster, and they've closely followed the outcomes of the children in the decades since.[32]

Project Ice Storm babies were born smaller and earlier than expected, especially if the storm occurred very early or very late in the pregnancy. As infants, they exhibited delays in cognitive and language development. When they were assessed at age five, the language and cognitive delays remained and they also showed increased rates of attention and behavioural problems. Ice Storm 'babies' are now teenagers and they're still showing the effects of their stressful start to life. In girls, prenatal maternal stress increased their risk of early puberty, obesity and asthma. In some children, their fingerprint patterns (a measure of developmental asymmetry typically seen in people with schizophrenia) are altered.

Overall, the boys tended to fare worse than the girls. King and her colleagues suggest some of this difference might have arisen from differences in the placenta, whereby the female placenta seems to provide protection against high levels of maternal stress hormones.

Project Ice Storm has shown how intimately an unborn child is connected to her mother. A mother's physical and emotional state profoundly impact in utero and childhood development.

'The implication of our research is the unborn child is more fragile and sensitive to the mother's environment than we thought,' says King. 'Our advice to mothers is to avoid or control stress if possible.' Of course, natural disasters can't be controlled or prevented, but King says that pregnant women and those supporting them should do whatever they can to limit their distress. We'll come back to this theme of stress and the vital role of social buffering time and time again during the book.

A newborn brain is a rough draft ready for editing

In 1928, Cajal wrote, 'at first, many imperfect connections are formed, and many errors of distribution occur ... but the incongruences are progressively corrected'. Cajal was right again. The processes of synapse formation, refinement and elimination provide a mechanism by which experiences, encoded as electrical signals, modify brain circuits both during prenatal development, childhood, the teenage years and well into adulthood.

The brain of our ready-to-be-born baby girl is about to be inscribed with the story of her life. Mother Nature has provided a rough draft. Her chapter outline is present, but the paragraphs, sentences and words, interwoven with the narrative, grammar and punctuation, will be written and rewritten, edited and continually revised over her lifespan.

In the next chapter, we'll take a look at what happens once our baby girl emerges from the womb into the world, where the roles of society and culture, parental expectations and beliefs, and personal experiences start to engender her brain.

2.

Childhood

IT WAS A DRIZZLY AUTUMNAL EVENING IN 2008 WHEN, TO MY dismay, my obstetrician perfunctorily stated, 'It's a boy'. I'd always had a strong feeling I was carrying a boy, so I wasn't disappointed I had a son. Instead, I was annoyed that after a night and day of hard labour the doctor took it upon himself to announce the sex of my firstborn, and in such a routine, offhand manner.

Nineteen months later and under the care of a different doctor, I had a single line written in my birth plan: 'Husband is to announce baby's sex.' After a shorter, easier second labour my second-born was hoisted above me. 'It's another boy!' I cried. 'I didn't say a word!' was the obstetrician's quick response. Luckily, my husband was too enthralled with his new son to mind that this time I made the call.

From the very moment a baby is born, the first words he or she will hear are usually 'it's a boy' or 'it's a girl'. Because human children are born into a gendered world, to understand development of the female human brain we have to understand the influence and expectations of gender.

In the last chapter, we looked at the influence of genes and hormones on brain development in utero. Assuming Mum is healthy, well nourished, buffers stress and can avoid toxins, biology is queen in determining how the brain grows in the cocoon of the womb. In this chapter, we'll consider how childhood brain development is a product of not only bottom-up biology, but complex social and environmental influences.

When we left off last chapter, an innate and exquisitely orchestrated process of neural folding, proliferation, migration, navigation and cell death had resulted in a 'rough draft' nervous system. When our newborn girl is catapulted from the protective environment of in utero life to the vibrant outside world, her brain is about a third of the size of an adult brain, and capable of coordinating only basic reflexes: suckling, crying, sleeping. From birth onwards, growth is extraordinary and the rough draft is sculpted and customised by her interaction with the world. During infancy, childhood and adolescence, life experiences – good and bad – leave their lasting imprints on the brain.

Brain development from birth to adulthood

Once upon a time, it was assumed brains stop growing by the time children started school. Evidence for this was based on post-mortem studies. To all appearances, 5-year-old and 45-year-old brains were identical. It wasn't until the advent of safe modern brain imaging that anyone felt able to peer inside children's skulls to see if this was true.[33]

Since the 1990s, MRI technologies have shown brain growth certainly is most rapid during the first few years of life, but development continues well beyond the kindergarten years. Catherine Lebel is a neuroscientist at the University of Calgary in Canada who uses various MRI techniques to chart brain development. She tells me her research tries to answer a very simple question: How does the brain change during childhood?

For one study, Lebel invited 103 children and young adults ranging in age from five to thirty to visit her lab. Each volunteer's brain was scanned using an advanced MRI technique called Diffusion Tensor Imaging (DTI) that gives unique information about brain microstructure. All volunteers were scanned at least twice about four years apart (some were scanned three or four times). The 221 scans charted how white and grey matter grew and changed over childhood, adolescence and into adulthood.

Lebel found that between ages five and thirty white matter volume increased while at the same time grey matter volume decreased. Because white-matter increases and grey-matter decreases offset one another, total brain volume didn't change much at all. [33, 34]

Although this particular study didn't look at brains older than thirty, numerous other imaging studies have found white matter volume continues to increase to a peak at about age fifty and is then gradually lost with normal ageing.[33, 35] Some witty folk have quipped that this reflects the morphological development of wisdom.[36] Grey matter loss slows down by the time we reach our twenties and the thickness of the cortex then stays reasonably stable until degeneration sets in with old age. Lebel's studies show the process of healthy brain development is orderly, follows a predictable pattern and tracks alongside the emergence of skills and behaviours. As brains get more organised, efficient and sophisticated, so too do the owners of those brains.

Taking a closer look at white and grey matter

If you closely examine a fresh slice of human brain or one of Lebel's DTI scans, you'll see two kinds of neural tissue: an outer folded layer of greyish–purple matter, and the underlying fibrous white matter.

Grey matter makes up the cortex and some deeper brain structures such as the amygdala and hippocampus (collectively called the limbic system). Grey matter contains cell bodies of neurons, their dendrites, and glia such as astrocytes.

White matter consists of axon bundles that connect different structures or parts of grey matter together. White matter tracts can be very short, span from the left to right hemisphere, or stretch down the spinal cord.

If you were to look down a microscope and zoom in on thin slices of white matter sliced from children's brains at different ages (or slices of rat brain, if that makes you feel more comfortable), you'd see the developmental modifications Lebel described often have little to do with the neurons themselves.

White matter modifications are due to oligodendrocytes, which extend long, thin, flattened processes that wrap round axons, like layer upon layer of protective cling film. The oligodendrocyte wraps are made of a fatty white substance called myelin that provides electrical insulation to axons and gives white matter its name. Changes in white matter volume therefore reflect how thickly wrapped axons are with myelin. This directly determines how well electrically insulated axons are, and thus how efficiently neurons are able to communicate. Quite simply, more myelin means faster communication.

As I mentioned in chapter 1, half of all neurons born in the developing brain die, but most cell death is complete before birth. Grey matter shrinkage during childhood and adolescence is mostly due to loss of superfluous synapses or connections between neurons.

While it seems like a terrible waste to kill off half of all newborn neurons and prune away half of the sprouting synapses, massive proliferation followed by removal is how the brain streamlines networks so it works more efficiently and adapts to the world we live in.

How do neurons choose their synaptic partners? And which synapses are retained and which are removed?

Professor Colin Akerman is a neuroscientist at Oxford University, and his research attempts to answer this question. Akerman and I shared the same ground-floor physiology lab during our PhD studies, and we caught up over coffee in the Department of Pharmacology in Oxford one rainy morning while I was writing this book. I asked how he describes 'synaptic matching'.

'The type, strength and distribution of synaptic connections determine the behaviour of individual neurons within a neural network,' he told me. 'These synaptic circuits develop through a combination of hardwired genetic mechanisms *and* plastic activity-dependent processes.' Nature, nurture or a bit of both, one might say.

'The decision is made in a "use it or lose it" fashion,' he says. 'Competitions take place between neural inputs, whereby some axons are more electrically active and "win" and those less active "lose" and get removed.'

When Akerman and I were students, the phrases 'cells that fire together, wire together' and 'synapses out of sync fail to link' were only just coming into common use. The two phrases are shorthand ways to describe how experience, in the form of neural activity, causes pre- and post-synaptic neurons to 'fire together' and 'wire together'. Synapse selection and elimination is coordinated by experience in a 'use it or lose it' fashion. Neural activity is the biological tool by which childhood experiences sculpt and streamline each individual brain.

Brain architecture is built by early experiences

Human babies are born far more immature than most species. Newborn gazelle stagger to their feet within moments of birth. We can barely stagger to our feet a year later. But as we're learning, this long, slow development is what makes us human, and we quickly outpace the gazelle.

Within her first two years, a baby learns to lift her head, sit, walk, run and climb. She loses her primitive grasping reflexes and learns to coordinate her hands to grab and feed herself, to hold a crayon and even draw a straight line. She learns to understand what is being said to her and to follow simple instructions, and begins to express herself using simple sentences, often with great conviction. Her personality – the unique set of psychological qualities that influence how she thinks, feels and behaves – begins to emerge.

By the time she starts school, she's a social little creature who is developing relationships separate from her immediate family. She has her own friends, temperament, likes and dislikes. She can tell stories, create art and is ready to learn to read, spell and do simple maths. Her capacity to think, problem solve, interact with others, show empathy and even develop a theory of mind (her awareness of others' states of mind) is emerging.

Children don't learn these skills in isolation. Every neural process, every thought, feeling and behaviour they develop, is embedded in and influenced by the world around them. Interaction with people, places and things is an absolute requirement for healthy brain development.

Children learn best by play. They're driven by an evolutionary urge to play, do, taste, explore, feel, smell, experiment and interact – with people and animals, pots and pans in the bottom drawer, and puddles of rain. It's by interacting so intensely with the world that their brains develop. Young brains are primed to learn and grow by experience, and the requirement for experience to refine synapses and develop skills is unconditional.

Our large, complex, social brains require a long experience-rich childhood to develop. It's been said our extended childhoods enable our brains to better match the rich experiences and diverse environments we humans inhabit. A long childhood is also the foundation of our mind and sense of self – those amorphous mental attributes that make each of us the devastatingly charming, adaptable and distinctive individuals we are.[37]

Young brains are plastic brains

Brain architecture is refined during periods of intense development known as critical periods. Most occur in infancy, but some arrive as late as the teenage years. During critical periods, brains rapidly develop abilities such as vision, language and social skills. Experience in the form of sensory input – vision, sound and so on – is required to form new synapses, strengthen existing connections, prune superfluous dendrites, and add more myelin when faster communication is required. Critical periods are when the brain not only uses but *absolutely requires* particular experiences to remodel and refine the rough draft circuits. The absence of the appropriate input during critical periods can be dire.

Consider children born with 'squint' (strabismus), a condition where the eyes do not look in the same direction. Normal development of depth perception requires both the left and right eye to work together in the first few months of life. Children with squint lack depth perception – they can't see in three dimensions or figure out how far away objects are.

Usually a squint self-corrects or is easily treated by wearing an eye-patch over the good eye. But if it persists or is left untreated, children can develop lazy eye (amblyopia), which is when the brain starts to ignore input from one of the eyes to avoid double vision. The earlier that treatment for squint starts the better, and there comes a point when the critical period for developing binocular vision closes (around age ten) and it becomes too late and too hard to treat.

Our adult brains are still capable of being changed by experience, but the effort required to change is greater. If you've recently tried to learn a musical instrument or language for the first time you'll be able to attest that learning is not impossible, but it is never as effortless as it would have been in childhood. This is for two reasons: critical periods have closed, and our overall capacity for brain plasticity is dialled down.

Opening and closing sensitive periods

Harvard neuroscientist Takao Hensch is curious about how and why plasticity waxes and wanes with age, and spends his time exploring the neural mechanisms responsible for the opening and closing of critical periods. He likens brain activity before the opening of a critical period to people in a concert hall all talking at once – noisy, unstructured and chaotic. It is only when the curtain opens that some semblance of structure is imposed on the haphazard chatter.

Hensch has found that two processes regulate critical period timing and 'calm the chattering crowd': development of neurons containing the inhibitory neurotransmitter GABA and molecular 'brakes'. Hensch is now busy working out how to control the timing of GABAergic inhibition and 'braking' in an effort to turn back the biological clock and reopen critical periods to correct early developmental problems.[38, 39]

Why have critical periods evolved? Why does the potential for plasticity dial down as we get older? You'd imagine it would be more beneficial to retain the infinite capacity for change in response to experience as we age. This might enable us to have unlimited potential to master new skills with ease, or overcome early childhood stress and trauma.

Most scholars agree it would be maladaptive to allow experience to trigger large-scale reorganisation in adult brains once skills have been learned and behaviours established. Our brains must 'stabilise' and start the job of processing the world around us instead of being continually modified by it. Hensch is cautious about the implications of reopening critical periods because an individual's basic identity is also shaped during these formative times. 'The earliest memories and experiences are essential in shaping character – and they profoundly influence everything that comes next,' he says. 'If rekindling plasticity is not undertaken with the utmost care, the rewiring of the brain could threaten to undermine one's sense of self.'[40]

Language acquisition in children – from universalist to specialist

Now we've peered down the lens of the microscope at what's happened to the brain during critical periods, let's zoom right out again and explore what happens to the human owners of developing brains. Of all the formative periods of intense learning and brain plasticity, human language is probably the easiest to conceptualise.

Babies learn language in two broad phases: first they understand words, then they speak. Babies begin babbling at around three months and start saying their first words around the age of one. By the time they're two they can say up to fifty words, easily understand hundreds more and by three they're able to use over 1000 words with adult-like sentence structure. This universal process of language acquisition occurs in all cultures and languages, which indicates its strongly neurobiological roots.

After puberty, we can still learn to understand and speak languages in addition to our native tongue, but it doesn't happen effortlessly. Unless we learn a language before puberty, we'll never be fully fluent or speak without an accent. This is because language is a skill best learned during a period of development when the language centres of the brain are most plastic.

The first year is a critical period for language acquisition, but it's worth pointing out that babies can hear what is happening from inside the womb by about the twenty-fourth to twenty-eighth week of gestation. Support for this comes from research showing that newborns display a slight preference for their mother's voice and for the language they hear in utero. Of course, babies are immersed in amniotic fluid and any sounds must be transmitted via the uterine wall, so what they hear is very muffled. Rather than learning any words, it's thought they get a sense of prosody or the patterns and rhythms of their mother's speech.[41]

If you were raising babies back in the mid 1990s, you might have come across the notion that playing classical music while your child was in utero would turn them into geniuses or at least guarantee a place at an Ivy League college. This was based on the research that babies could hear and respond to music in the womb. Clearly some parents thought there was no point in foetuses wasting time floating round in amniotic fluid when they could get a head start on their education.

There is no compelling evidence for the so-called Mozart Effect (and no evidence of harm, except to bank accounts), yet the idea is catchy and there remains a market for prenatal music lessons and equipment. One device I came upon when browsing online is the Babypod, 'an intra-vaginal speaker designed to broadcast music inside the womb to an unborn baby'. Hmmm.

Whether they've heard vaginally broadcast symphonies or simply been soothed more naturally by their mother's muffled voice, all babies are born as 'citizens of the world' or 'language universalists'.

Patricia Kuhl, a professor of speech and hearing science at the University of Washington, coined these phrases and her research shows that babies in every corner of the globe are totally equivalent in their ability to discriminate all the sounds of all languages at birth. Adults and older children can't do this. By our first birthday we become 'culture-bound listeners' and can only discriminate the sounds of our native language, and not those of foreign tongues.[42]

Take, for example, the language development in a baby born in Tokyo versus a baby born in London. At birth, both are language universalists, but their parents are likely 'culture-bound'. Native Japanese-speaking parents will find it hard to distinguish between *r* and *l* sounds; both sounds are perceived as *r*. If the Japanese and English infants were tested at six months of age, both babies could easily distinguish between *r* and *l*, but by ten months of age the Japanese infants would lose the distinction because they don't hear those sounds spoken during this sensitive phase. Similarly, Spanish speakers distinguish between the words *pano* and *bano*, whereas English speakers treat the *p* and *b* sounds of these words the same.

Given that many languages use identical sounds, infants must learn how to take meaning in from language. During the first year of life the 'universalist' infant becomes specialised and 'tunes in' to their native frequency. The pattern follows for bilingual babies too – they simply become tuned in to the sounds of two different languages.

Children don't learn language by sitting down and memorising vocab lists and rules of grammar. Learning doesn't require formal teaching or effort, but it does require warm, engaged adults who actively talk and engage with the baby.

If you talk to a baby you'll find you automatically use a higher pitch, slow your tempo, exaggerate your intonation and facial expressions: '*Hiiiiii baby, do I love you, do I love youuuuu? Yeeees, yes I do.*' Babies prefer listening to this type of speech; they don't want or need to be spoken to as adults. This type of interaction has been called 'motherese' (although the term 'parent-ese' is rightfully being used, as fathers do it too) or 'serve and return' learning. Similar to a game of ping-pong, adults and children interact by cooing, babbling, making facial expressions, and chattering back and forth.

Deprivation during the first year – a critical period for language

Two groups of children have shown us this absolute requirement for the language critical period: children who are born deaf, and those who grow up in isolation or deprivation without 'serve and return' interactions.[41]

Being born deaf in the days before hearing aids, cochlear implants and newborn screening meant growing up with severe learning difficulties. Deaf children struggled with vocabulary, grammar and syntax (the set of rules, principles and processes that govern the sentence structure, such as the order of words). Deaf children also lacked the non-verbal aspects of conversation such as turn-taking, asking for clarification, eye contact and greetings. They had trouble learning to read, and struggled with maths and other higher-order cognitive skills. Around eight months is the end of the critical period in which a hearing device has to be fitted for deaf children to develop similar cognitive skills as their hearing playmates.[43]

Interestingly, deaf children who are exposed to sign language (often because they're born to deaf parents) don't develop the same learning problems. Sign language is thought to be their 'native tongue' and deaf babies are even seen 'babbling' with their hands as early as six months.

Readers will be familiar with the horrors reported in Romania in the late 1980s following the fall of Romania's Communist dictator Nicolae Ceauşescu. Thousands of children were found abandoned in orphanages not only half starved but socially and emotionally deprived. British families adopted many of these orphans and their outcomes have since been tracked and compared with adoptees from within the UK who didn't experience deprivation. In 2017 a landmark research paper was published in *The Lancet* describing 165 adoptees who are now in their mid to late twenties.[44]

Compared to the British-adoptee control group, more Romanian adoptees experienced low educational achievement and unemployment, and were far more likely to seek help from mental health services; many were diagnosed with depression and anxiety, which emerged during their teenage years. They had problems with attention, disinhibited social engagement and symptoms of autism. One protective element appears to be spending less than six months in orphanages – these adults were no different from UK adoptees. The authors concluded 'severe adversity, occurring because of institutional deprivation in early childhood, can have a profound and lasting psychological impact despite subsequent environmental enrichment in well-resourced and supportive families.' We now understand warm nurturing relationships in infancy are *absolutely critical* for healthy brain development.

Toxic stress in childhood leaves lasting effects on the brain

'It's possible we've underestimated the importance of childhood,' says Professor Richie Poulton, head of the Dunedin Study, a research program that has closely tracked every aspect of the lives of 1037 people born in Dunedin, New Zealand in 1972 and 1973.

Early life experiences shape developing brain architecture and strongly affect whether children grow up to be healthy, productive members of society. During early childhood, enhanced brain plasticity is a double-edged sword: increased opportunity for learning is paired with increased vulnerability to deprivation and stress. Toxic stress is defined as stress that is extreme or long lasting or occurs outside an environment of supportive, attached caregiver relationships. Toxic stress derails brain development, with damaging effects on learning, behaviour, and physical and mental health across the lifespan.[45] This vulnerability is clearly demonstrated by the Dunedin Study.

Poulton has been able to predict with reasonable accuracy which children will grow up with social or health problems. Growing up in a socioeconomically deprived family, exposure to maltreatment, low IQ and poor self-control are proven predictors of poor adult health and social outcomes including criminal convictions, prescription fills, welfare claims and hospital visits. This 'high cost' group of adults could be reliably identified by three years of age. Rather than blaming the victim for economic burden following on from childhood disadvantage, Poulton suggests we focus on early-years intervention or what he calls 'grey-matter infrastructure' so we can lift health and social wellbeing as disadvantaged children grow up.[46]

Another 'natural experiment' – the Christchurch earthquakes

Another group of children living a few hours north of Dunedin in New Zealand have given us additional insights into how extreme stress in infancy impacts social, emotional and cognitive development in childhood.

Starting in September 2010, my hometown of Christchurch was hit by a series of massive earthquakes. The most devastating was on 22 February 2011, when 185 people died and 6600 people were injured. Everyone, including my family, was deeply affected. Over the next two years there were 14 000 aftershocks, including thirty-two earthquakes over magnitude five. Friends of mine took to playing 'guess the size' on Facebook, and many were able to determine the fault line and magnitude within decimal-point accuracy. People called living with continual shaking, damaged infrastructure, insurance battles and unrelenting psychological stress 'the new normal'.

In the past few years I've started hearing stories of Christchurch schools struggling with large numbers of children starting school with learning difficulties and behavioural problems. For example, I knew of one class of twenty-two children that required four extra learning support teachers. There was a general consensus among my friends and family this was the impact of children growing up in 'the new normal'.

In much the same way the Montreal Ice Storm babies have been tracked, a cohort of Christchurch children are now being followed by researcher Kathleen Liberty, an associate professor of child development at the University of Canterbury. I met with Liberty in her office just after Christmas 2016 to discuss what she calls her 'post-EQ children'.

In New Zealand, children begin school on the day of or near to their fifth birthday, and Liberty has been gathering data on the social, emotional and cognitive development of these new entrants since 2006. After the earthquakes she has been able to revisit the same primary schools and gather data on post-EQ children then compare them to the 'old normal' baseline.

Liberty confirms there are significantly more behavioural problems and post-traumatic stress symptoms in the children who started school after experiencing the earthquakes. In her 2016 paper, published in *PLOS Natural Disasters*, she reports twenty-one per cent of post-EQ children showed six or more post-traumatic symptoms such as being withdrawn, clingy, irritable, defiant, unhappy or having sudden changes of mood (six or more symptoms is highly indicative of post-traumatic stress disorder, PTSD, in children). Less than nine per cent of pre-EQ children showed as many symptoms.[47]

One of the strongest predictors of whether children would experience difficulties was the age the child was when the earthquakes began. Surprisingly, children younger than two when the sequence began were more vulnerable than older children. But Liberty suggests this is because the older children experienced a buffer period of normal stress-free brain development. She guesses older children possessed the behaviours, language and cognitive skills to communicate with parents and perhaps make some sense of what was happening when the room was shaking, people were screaming and the world was literally falling down around them.

Because earthquakes strike without warning, the post-EQ boys and girls have grown up in an unpredictable world, many in highly stressed families. During a period of incredible neural plasticity, the children's stress response systems were activated thousands of times. Exposure to extreme stress before the age of two activates the immature stress response system including the hypothalamus-pituitary-adrenal (HPA) axis and brain regions that regulate its activity, with enduring consequences for children's behaviour.[48, 49]

You'll no doubt be wondering if there were sex differences in how children reacted to the quakes. Liberty told me that sex differences weren't detected. Primary-school-age boys and girls were equally affected by growing up with earthquake stress. However, a study of 525 Christchurch teenagers six months after the earthquakes reported clear sex differences in the development of PTSD. Only thirteen per cent of boys showed clinically significant PTSD symptoms compared to thirty-four per cent of teenage girls. This finding is consistent with other disaster zone research and PTSD research in general that finds higher prevalence of PTSD amongst post-pubertal girls and women compared to boys and men.[50]

Intriguingly, one of the buffers against distress was being part of a Maori community. Other researchers have also found the social connectedness, spiritual support and collective dynamics associated within the indigenous community contributed to the resilience of the Maori children in Christchurch.[51]

Liberty tells me she is now working with schools and families to help children learn to regulate and understand their own emotions and to build resilience. One myth she is working hard to dispel is that parents, in particular the mother, are to blame for how resilient or stressed children are. 'Children are *not* having problems because of how Mum reacts during an earthquake,' she says. 'Mothers don't cause the problems. The earthquakes did,' she said. 'But parents are in a unique position to teach their children how to manage their stress response.'

Are resilient children born or made?

In every study I've described, including the Ice Storm babies and the Dunedin Study, a proportion of each cohort displayed exceptional resilience and flourished despite the circumstances. Nearly thirty per cent of the post-EQ children in Christchurch showed no symptoms of post-traumatic stress. One in five Romanian orphans are completely unaffected by their maltreatment. These resilient children are the ones who can give us unique insights into opportunities for early-years 'grey-matter infrastructure' support and intervention.

It's important to consider stress and resilience from a bottom-up, outside-in, top-down perspective. Family ties and psychological coping mechanisms strengthen resilience, but resilience also has biological roots.

All children differ in their biological susceptibility to life experiences in a 'for better and for worse' manner. Some kids are particularly sensitive to both highly stressful *and* highly nurturing environments. Like orchids, such children bloom if lovingly cultivated, but wilt and wither if neglected. In contrast, adaptable resilient children who don't get easily stressed are like little dandelions: they'll grow and thrive anywhere. Studies are now showing that 'orchid' genes linked to particular enzymes or brain chemical receptors, if and only if combined with early childhood toxic stress, can trigger behavioural problems and mood disorders later in life. We'll come back to this intriguing concept in chapter 6 when we look at mental health.

Experiences of gender

Because experiences build the brain, we can't consider female brain development without reflecting on the experiences of girlhood. As Cordelia Fine has pointed out, society places considerable weight on biological sex, and gender socialisation of boys and girls starts at birth. Life-long brain plasticity has been demonstrated in response to experiences as varied as learning language and music, emotional regulation, taxi driving and even juggling. There is little doubt early childhood experiences of what it means to be a girl will also make an impression on brain architecture.

Boys and girls go out to play

Walking through my sons' primary school, I can very nearly divide the senior playground in half by gender. In one half, roaming herds of nine-, ten-, and eleven-year-old same-sex peers play competitive ball games replete with complex rules that are debated and challenged constantly for 'fairness'. Wandering between the ball games are same-sex clusters of twos or threes chatting, whispering and peeling off to regularly seek approval or intervention from a teacher. If you've ever observed primary school children left to their own devices, you'll have no trouble guessing which group is girls and which is boys.

I'm a mother of two boys in the roaming herd, but my memories of girlhood are clear. I rarely roamed with the ball-chasing herd; rather, I spent my time whispering secrets, forming and breaking alliances, and giggling with my girlfriends till I nearly wet my pants. And according to my mother, I regularly reported in to her about who was saying what to whom and why they shouldn't and what I'd like her to do about it.

Highly respected gender researcher Professor Melissa Hines, Director of the Gender Development Research Centre at the University of Cambridge, has summarised the differences in play shown by boys and girls during childhood.[52] Hines claims that long before children reach school age it is possible to predict with a reasonable degree of certainty who is a boy and who is a girl by the toys they choose and the friends they play with. (That d-value statistic I introduced you to in the introduction is around 0.80 for toy choice and playmate preference.)[53]

Between the ages of one and two, children are very flexible in their thinking about gender – a little girl might firmly believe she'll grow up to be a man like Dad, she'll happily play with boys and girls, and won't show a strong preference for 'girls toys'. By about age two children become very motivated to relate to other members of their 'group', girls with girls, boys with boys, and they often become very strict about adhering to gender stereotypes: 'Girls are princesses who wear pink' is the classic example. (I remember being mystified when at the same age my eldest son would refuse to even let me dry him with a pink towel after his bath. Now I understand this was developmentally normal!) Despite the best attempts at gender-neutral parenting, parents report that girls will often prefer to play with dolls and boys will prefer to play with cars and weapons. Groups of boys or brothers are also more likely to play 'rough-and-tumble' physical games.

Gender difference in play and friend preference is seen across cultures and continues into the school years, although girls tend to relent a little and will happily choose more traditional 'boy toys' such as Lego if playing alone. Boys, on the other hand, only get more stringent in their choices (this is thought to be because of the pressures some of them face to be 'little men').

There are two broad theories explaining these sex differences in toy preference, playmate choice and play style: nature and nurture (surprised?). Many people feel uncomfortable looking at the biological roots of gender, and as Margaret McCarthy notes it is the 'collision of gender and biology that generates the most heat in the debate about the female brain'.

Hormones and the 'mini puberty' of infancy

Boys and girls do differ a tiny bit during infancy. The *average* newborn girl is ever so slightly smaller, less fussy, easier to soothe and more socially aware than the *average* boy. Her language, memory and motor skills also track slightly ahead during the first year. Part of this may be due to the effects of testosterone early in gestation that masculinise or feminise certain regions of the brain.[11] Another reason may be 'mini puberty'. Technically it's called the 'postnatal endocrine surge' but, like 'puberty proper', it's when testosterone and oestrogen are released from testes and ovaries.

The hypothalamic-pituitary-gonadal (HPG) axis develops and is active during the first half of pregnancy. During the second half of pregnancy, hormones from the placenta switch the axis into silent mode. In girls, once the effects of placental and maternal hormones have worn off the axis brake is released and it jolts into action for a while. A week or so after birth the ovaries start manufacturing oestrogen, causing slight swelling of the breasts and growth of the uterus. In infant boys testosterone causes penis and testes growth, and sebaceous gland and acne development.[54]

Mini-puberty is complete by the age of two and the HPG axis stays quiet till 'puberty proper'. What this means in terms of brain development is unknown; however, neuroscientist Lise Eliot, author of *Pink Brain, Blue Brain*, speculates that just as prenatal hormones organise the brain, the postnatal surge in hormones might create a critical period for nudging infant brain development further down the male or female trajectory.[11]

One clue that hormones influence toy and playmate choice comes from studies of non-human primates. Given the large effects of cultural and societal expectations on human children, primates are important model species for investigating the biology of sex differences. In a review for the *Journal of Neuroscience Research*, Elizabeth Lonsdorf summarises sex differences in primates that echo differences found in human children.

She points out that male primates spend more time in 'rough-and-tumble' play, and they roam further from their mothers than their sisters do. Females groom others more than males in the first year of life, and perform a specific behaviour called 'stick carrying,' in which a stick is cradled and carried in a form of play mothering. Lonsdorf concludes that gender socialisation in humans magnifies the differences between boys and girls, but primate studies suggest 'these behavioral sex differences are rooted in our biological and evolutionary heritage'.[55]

Gender stereotypes begin before birth

'Cars and trucks or ribbons and bows. What are we having? We're about to know!'

Thanks to technology we no longer need to wait until the bub arrives to deploy colour-coded gender stereotyping. It can begin in the womb. In a trend unique to the social media age, gender-reveal parties are now a 'thing'. For the uninitiated reader, parents-to-be host gender-reveal parties for friends and family with the purpose of announcing whether they're having a baby boy or girl, and the parties take place months before the baby is born.

A scroll through Pinterest shows some very creative ways to announce whether the unborn babe is a boy or girl. The most popular methods seem to be encouraging guests to simultaneously bite into pink or blue cupcakes covered in gender-neutral icing, opening giant boxes filled with pink or blue helium balloons, or smashing open piñatas filled with pink or blue confetti. Beforehand, guests are invited to bet on the outcome, or cast a vote for 'Team Pink' or 'Team Blue'.

Because 'gender disappointment' is real, I hate to think what happens if the cut cake isn't the desired shade of pastel. Do mothers hoping for a little girl but faced with a box of blue balloons hide their grief till their guests go home?

Clearly I'm cynical about this trend. And I'm not the only one. Many feminists have expressed concern that gender-reveal parties are, by default, celebrating and reinforcing gender stereotypes for the unborn child.

Whether they intend to or not, parents respond to baby boys and baby girls differently, including in utero. Mothers who know they're carrying a baby boy will claim their boy's movements to be far more active or vigorous compared to mothers carrying girls. Studies of whether foetal movement can predict sex are contradictory. One careful study from the Netherlands monitored 123 women, fifty-six of whom were carrying baby boys and sixty-seven baby girls. Foetal movements, heart rate and heart rate variability were assessed, and researchers concluded there were no sex differences in movement.[56]

Once babies are born all bets are off, and even those parents who swear they're raising their children in a gender-neutral manner find it hard to be 'neutral' all the time. For example, mothers of daughters use more 'emotion' words than mothers of sons (e.g. 'love', 'scared', 'worried', 'pleased', 'cross', etc.). By the time the daughters start talking they use more emotion words than their brothers.[57]

Lise Eliot posits that boys and girls enter the world with slight differences and how parents react to those differences (based on unconscious biases or explicit beliefs) contribute to what can grow into troublesome gaps. 'Some parents maintain traditional gender stereotypes and expectations,' she says. This may 'nurture' the 'nature', so to speak.[11]

It's easy to forget that parents aren't the only social influence on children. As discussed above, the primary schoolyard is fairly segregated down gender lines. Researchers theorise that the 'self-imposed segregation' may cause children to develop two cultures, each with different norms for interaction. Within these boy or girl groupings, children self-socialise and reinforce ideas about how boys and girls should play, react and speak. Together children 'practise' gendered behaviours. As a result girls become more 'girl-like' and boys more 'boy-like'.[58, 59]

Why do expectations of gender matter?

For some reason, our obsession with sex differences is particularly pervasive when it comes to educating our children. Neurobiologist Donna Maney has compiled a list of claims commonly presented to teachers in professional development workshops in the USA.

Some of the spurious claims include 'the female brain is more active than the male brain, which often goes into a pause state after tasks. To break the pause, boys must use loud voices, run or jump,' and 'boys have less oxytocin than girls, which makes them uncomfortable with eye contact, so they should be seated side-by-side'.[60]

One boys' high school website claims that boys have less serotonin in their brains than girls, which means they are more likely to act impulsively and be less able to sit still for long periods of time. You'd be forgiven for thinking it was time to reclassify both serotonin and oxytocin as classroom seating-plan chemicals!

Why does it matter if parents and teachers have expectations of gender?

It matters deeply if expectations become stereotypes. Gender stereotypes refer to particular attributes believed to characterise boys or girls as separate groups (e.g. girls can sit still, boys can't). Stereotypes inherently ignore within-group differences (some girls can't sit still, and some boys are great at sitting) and exaggerate between-group differences.

Around the world men believe they are smarter and more brilliant than women. A study of twelve countries, including Australia, Britain and the US, published in the *British Journal of Psychology*, found 'male hubris' and 'female humility' in self-estimates of intelligence (which weren't aligned with actual IQ).[61]

This destructive gender stereotype emerges in childhood. A study published in *Science* in 2017 found that six-year-old girls have already absorbed gendered beliefs about intelligence despite there being exactly zero difference in academic ability. Girls believe 'brilliance, giftedness and genius' are male qualities. In the study, little girls were less interested in games they perceived as meant for 'really, really smart kids'. They went from being enthusiastic about playing 'smart-kid' games at ages four and five to saying, 'This isn't the game for me,' around age six. Boys of the same age didn't hold the same beliefs. It gets worse: the six-year-old girls happily grouped boys into the 'children who are really, really smart' category, but not their own gender.[62]

What do growing brains need to thrive?

It seems like I've spent much of this chapter exploring what can go wrong during childhood – from the effects of toxic stress to learning negative gender stereotypes. If you have young children you're probably ready to drop the book and run off to bulk-buy cotton wool and bubble wrap. Given what we know about normal and abnormal brain development, what experiences do infants and children (the dandelions *and* the orchids) need to thrive, not just survive? What can adults who raise children do to foster healthy, happy brains?

Faced with wading through more childhood development literature in search of an answer, I instead picked up the phone and called my friend and colleague Dr Kristy Goodwin. Goodwin is a children's learning and development researcher and she has summarised seven essential experiences or, as she calls them, 'building blocks' for optimal brain development.

These common-sense building blocks include:

- ♀ **Attachments and relationships.** Warm, predictable and loving relationships allow children to feel secure, safe and unstressed.
- ♀ **Language.** Infants and young children need ample opportunities to hear and use language: 'serve-and-return' interactions are crucial.
- ♀ **Sleep.** Sleep is vital for children's emotional, physical and mental development.
- ♀ **Play.** Through play, babies and children develop cognitive skills, creativity and emotional regulation. They need opportunities to experiment and explore, including time outdoors in nature. Goodwin highlights the modern-day need to counteract 'screen time' with 'green time'.
- ♀ **Physical movement.** Children need to master simple then complex motor skills in order to develop more sophisticated, higher-order thinking skills later on.
- ♀ **Nutrition.** Quality nutrition is vital for optimal development. Children's diets need to be rich in foods that contain essential fatty acids optimal for brain development.
- ♀ **Executive function skills.** Children need to master simple higher-order thinking skills such as impulse control and working memory.[63]

'Given that we know experience accounts for about seventy per cent of a child's development,' says Goodwin, 'it's critical that we provide them with the right types of experiences.' Goodwin and I agree that childhood is a very sacred time. It's a unique period in the lifespan that needs to be treasured, nurtured and protected.

3.

Puberty

PUBERTY IS A RITE OF PASSAGE MOST OF US READING THIS BOOK will have passed through. If you're a woman, maybe you have fond memories of shopping for your first bra, and like me you were excitedly anticipating the arrival of your first period. Or perhaps your transition was full of angst, confusion or humiliation.

As Kaz Cooke writes in *Girl Stuff*, puberty is when you get bigger, fluffier, leakier and moodier. It's also when the potential for embarrassment goes through the roof. I concur with Cooke that the capacity for embarrassment crashes back down to earth once you enter adulthood.

Every girl follows her own individual pathway through puberty – some grow breasts before pubic hair, others sprout underarm hair years before their first period. Some girls start maturing early, around age eight, progress rapidly and have their first period about age ten. Others blossom later and travel slowly.

Puberty isn't only about the physical changes. It involves the beginning of neurodevelopmental, emotional and behavioural changes unlike any seen since infancy. As you'll learn, there are other outside-in and top-down elements that influence what happens to girls during puberty besides hormones.

From an evolutionary perspective, puberty is all about getting the body and brain ready to date, mate and nurture offspring. In both boys and girls, it begins with the activation of the hypothalamic-pituitary-gonadal (HPG) axis, which results in:

- ♀ Maturation of gametes (oocytes/eggs in the ovaries of girls, spermatozoa in the testes of boys).
- ♀ Increased levels of sex hormones (ovarian hormones in girls; testicular hormones in boys) and adrenal hormones (in both boys and girls).
- ♀ Appearance of secondary sex characteristics (breasts etc. in girls; larger penis, testicles and muscles in boys).
- ♀ Fertility (menstrual cycle in girls, ability to ejaculate in boys).

Puberty results in the maturation of a body capable of reproduction, but the physical changes of puberty alone aren't enough to fertilise an egg. The phase of adolescence results in the maturation of the social, emotional and cognitive skills required to ensure the sperm and egg get the chance to meet in the first place.

From a neurobiological perspective, we can think of puberty as the second sensitive phase for hormone-driven brain development. Alongside prenatal life and infancy, puberty is when brain architecture is extra sensitive to sex hormones. I like to think of puberty as 'finishing school' for the brain. It's when neural circuits laid down in utero and during infancy are refined and then activated.

Many of the same neural mechanisms involved in early development get in on the act again: neurogenesis and the elaboration and pruning of synapses and dendrites.

When considering this two-phase brain development concept, keep in mind that during the first wave of hormone-dependent sculpting, ovarian hormones played no role in female brain development (unlike the male brain, which was sculpted by testosterone). Puberty is when ovarian hormones finally come to the fore.

Hormones are only one piece of the puzzle, and a pubertal girl's brain and her thoughts, feelings and behaviours are profoundly influenced by the world around her, including by gender, culture, education, family environment and shifting friendship groups. Her brain continues to experience neuroplastic change well into her twenties.

In this chapter we'll take a look at the neural control of puberty, and focus on the earliest stages of adolescence. In the next chapter we'll consider the neurobiology of the menstrual cycle, and finally in chapter 5 we'll explore the teenage brain.

First puberty

The tween growth spurt is one of the more obvious and least intimate signs of puberty. Breast development (thelarche), pubic hair growth (pubarche), armpit hair growth, and the arrival of monthly periods (menarche) are the others. But the first hormonal changes sending a child towards adulthood commence far earlier than most people realise, somewhere between the ages of six and eight. Adrenarche (yes, another *arche* – pronounced *arky* and Greek for 'origins' or 'new beginnings') refers to the awakening of the adrenal glands, which sit atop the kidneys.

The adrenal glands are made up of two parts: the adrenal medulla that secretes the hormones adrenaline and noradrenaline (known as epinephrine and norepinephrine in the US) and the adrenal cortex, which manufactures three types of hormones – mineralcorticoids, glucocorticoids and androgens. Androgens include testosterone, and the androgen precursor molecule dehydroepiandrosterone (DHEA). Androgens are what we might typically think of as 'male' hormones. But girls make them too.

Normal maturation of the adrenal glands in both boys and girls results in development of pubic hair, underarm hair, adult body odour and the dreaded acne. The mechanisms that initiate 'puberty proper' – breasts and periods – involve a different hormonal cascade, which we'll get into shortly. This means occasionally a healthy girl as young as seven or eight can sprout a few pubic hairs or require deodorant to mask underarm odour, but she isn't necessarily on track to get her period early or develop breasts. The early signs of adrenarche don't indicate precocious puberty.[64]

Let's take a closer look at adrenarche, because it's increasingly recognised as an important phase of childhood development. Dr Lisa Mundy is the project coordinator of a longitudinal study of puberty in Australia, the Childhood to Adolescence Transition Study (CATS). CATS is interested in what gives children a healthy start to adolescence with a special focus on adrenarche.[65-68]

Mundy and her team have followed over 1200 children from ages eight or nine through adolescence, and at the time of writing, some have embarked on their second year of high school. The CATS team have overturned the idea that ages surrounding adrenarche are a developmentally 'quiet' time for children, one when we can simply practise benign neglect.

Instead, adrenarche has significant implications for children's social and emotional wellbeing long before 'puberty proper' begins. One of the most surprising findings to emerge from Mundy's research has been the discovery that rising levels of adrenal androgens impact emotion and behaviour. In particular, early adrenarche is associated with greater risk of mental health symptoms.[69] High DHEA levels predicted problems, but girls and boys respond quite differently.

'We looked at DHEA and we found higher levels in boys were associated with emotional and behaviour problems,' Mundy told me. 'The same association wasn't there for girls. Instead we found DHEA was linked to social problems with their friends.'

Child and adolescent psychiatrist Professor George Patton, a colleague of Mundy, believes it is time to pay much closer attention to the social and emotional development of children in these age groups. 'Benign neglect worked back in the 1950s when social structures and communities were in place to support kids,' he told me over the phone. 'The world is a lot less understandable and predictable than it used to be.'

The HPO axis – how the brain and body talk puberty

Popular wisdom would have you think puberty begins in the ovaries and a young body suddenly steeped in oestrogen grows curvaceous and fecund. Whilst 'puberty proper' involves the gonads and is called (as you might have guessed) gonadarche, it all begins in the brain.

To understand the neurobiological underpinnings of puberty, we need to return to the HPO axis, the trio that unites body and brain and orchestrates our reproductive lives.

In brief, the HPO axis works like this:

- ♀ Hypothalamus signals to the pituitary gland via the gonadotropin-releasing hormone (GnRH).
- ♀ GnRH causes release of luteinising hormone (LH) and follicle-stimulating hormone (FSH).
- ♀ LH and FSH stimulate the ovaries to release oestrogens and progesterone.
- ♀ Oestrogen and progesterone exert their wide-ranging effects on the body and brain.
- ♀ LH, FSH, oestrogen and progesterone signal back to the hypothalamus and pituitary, forming complex positive and negative feedback loops.

Awakening the biological clock

During our fertile years between puberty and menopause GnRH is secreted from a pulse generator in the hypothalamus in a rhythmic fashion. I like to think of it as the neural manifestation of the famed biological clock – *tick-tick-tick*.

In childhood GnRH is released, but instead of a rhythmic *tick-tick-tick*, the release is a low, slow and continuous *whrrrr*. This low-level steady release maintains the HPO axis in a sort of 'hormonal hibernation', an event unique to humans and a few higher-order primates. Hormonal hibernation means humans have a prolonged childhood and the requisite phases of brain development, socialisation and learning. Mother Nature seems to know a little girl is in no way capable of bearing and caring for another human, so she makes it impossible for her to bring a baby into the world until she's mature enough to cope. Although, it goes without saying, menarche doesn't necessarily indicate she's ready either!

Nomenclature often gives clues about the roles of hormones and the job of GnRH in the pituitary is clearly indicated by its title – it releases gonadotropin hormones. The two main gonadotropins are FSH and LH, and thanks to their hypothalamic conductor they too are released in a rhythmic *tick-tick-tick* from the pituitary. FSH, as the name suggests, stimulates the growth of follicles in the ovary, promotes development of the egg, and causes secretion of oestradiol (the main type of oestrogen). LH is responsible for causing the follicle to rupture, triggering ovulation.

LH and FSH are produced in varying amounts throughout the lifespan. During childhood levels are low, but at puberty LH secretion increases until it surges to reach levels twenty to forty times greater than in early girlhood. FSH secretion, meanwhile, increases two- to three-fold. FSH won't overtake LH again until after menopause when, unchecked by ageing ovaries, both levels skyrocket.

Because the brain contains oestrogen receptors, oestrogen can influence how we think, feel and behave. One striking example of this is seen at menopause, when fluctuating levels of ovarian hormones cause hot flashes, night sweats, mood swings and forgetfulness. Once hormones level out in the years after a woman's last menstrual period, the symptoms disappear too.

Progesterone is another hormone produced by the ovaries, more specifically in the corpus luteum, which develops from the follicle after it bursts, releasing the egg at ovulation. Progesterone and oestrogen work synergistically. For example, pubertal breast development requires oestrogen to prime the cells and progesterone causes cell differentiation and growth. There aren't as many receptors for progesterone in the brain as there are for oestrogens, but it's becoming clearer it too can regulate thinking, mood and neuroplasticity, and may even play a role in recovery from brain injury.

Awakening the clock with a genetic KISS

What exactly awakens the GnRH biological clock? Is there an internal calendar marking the years? Or are there 'outside-in' elements that influence the timing of puberty, such as nutrition, the environment or family dynamics?

Genes largely determine when a girl will start to blossom. We surmise this is because girls, their mothers and sisters all experience menarche at around the same age. Studies have shown heritability ranges from fifty per cent to eighty per cent. After reading this statistic, I Skyped my mum to find out how old she was when she got her first period. She remembers being about twelve and half – the same as me. My sister texted that she was a week shy of twelve. Puberty timing in mothers is also reflected in the timing of onset of puberty in their sons.[70]

The gene responsible for awakening GnRH neurons is the rather whimsically named KISS-1, which is expressed in a small cluster of neurons in the pulse generator of the hypothalamus. KISS-1 codes for a protein called kisspeptin, which is released from neurons with two other peptide hormones, neurokinin B and dynorphin; the trio are popularly referred to as KNDy (pronounced 'candy').

There is a story behind these sweet-sounding names. KISS-1 was discovered by Danny Welch, a melanoma researcher, when he was working at Penn State College of Medicine in the town of Hershey. He named the new gene KISS-1 in honour of the Hershey's Kisses made at the town's famous chocolate factory.

No-one had any idea KISS-1 was involved in puberty until an unusual family approached reproductive endocrinologist

Stephanie Seminara, who runs the Reproductive Endocrine Unit at Massachusetts General Hospital. In the early 2000s a large family in which three marriages were between first cousins came to Seminara's clinic hoping for treatment. There were nineteen children in the family and of these six (four men and two women) suffered from a form of abnormal puberty called idiopathic hypogonadotropic hypogonadism (IHH). IHH is characterised by abnormal or absent GnRH pulses, so puberty doesn't start. It's rare, but the disorder provided Seminara's team a unique opportunity to look at the control of GnRH in humans. The family underwent genetic testing, and it was found that the gene for the kisspeptin receptor was mutated. This meant kisspeptin couldn't act on GnRH neurons to switch on puberty.[71]

Although Seminara didn't know it at the time, a group from the INSERM in Paris used a similar approach in another IHH family. In this instance, a twenty-year-old man was referred to Nicholas de Roux's clinic with symptoms of delayed puberty. He had an abnormally small penis and testes, short stature and sparse pubic hair. It turned out that three of his four brothers had similar traits; and one of his sisters, who was sixteen, had partially developed breasts and had only ever had one period. Their parents were first cousins who progressed normally through puberty and were clearly fertile. Again, genetic screening revealed that the receptor for kisspeptin was faulty.[72] Thanks to these families, kisspeptin's pivotal role in the neuroendocrine control of reproduction was established. Since its discovery, roles for kisspeptin have been found for ovulation, embryo implantation, development of the placenta, pregnancy and childbirth, and in 2017 it was implicated in menopausal hot flashes.

Is puberty starting at younger ages?

IHH and delayed puberty are relatively rare, but it seems like we're all getting more familiar with stories about early puberty. No-one is comfortable hearing about five-year-old girls shopping for a bra, or learning to manage a period at the same time as navigating kindergarten. Of course, the media hypes the stories and they're often told in the same breath as stories of nineteenth-century girls not starting their periods until they were seventeen.

Are the girls of today really starting puberty nearly a decade younger than previous centuries, and even earlier than girls in the 1960s? My GP said she's convinced this is the case, and so were plenty of other experts I spoke to. But there are some nuances to the story.

Girls are reaching puberty earlier than they used to, confirms Jayashri Kulkarni, a professor of psychiatry at Monash University. 'But while it's true that girls are experiencing some pubertal changes earlier on – developing breasts, for instance – the actual age they get their first period has actually stabilised at around thirteen years,' she explains. Data from the US confirms this: girls are getting their first period on average four to six months younger than girls did in previous centuries. But they are developing breasts up to two years earlier.

Marcia Herman-Giddens, an adjunct professor and paediatrician at the University of North Carolina, first recorded this finding. In the 80s and 90s she was seeing more and more girls coming to her clinic with signs of early puberty. This observation worried her, so she coordinated a number of nationwide studies looking at the average ages girls began puberty and compared the timing to previous generations.

Her initial finding was that the average age for the onset of breast development was eight years and nine months for African American girls, nine years three months for Hispanic girls, and nine years eight months for Caucasian and Asian American girls.[73] Subsequent studies in the United States confirmed that today's girls are developing breasts earlier than in previous generations.[74] The same pattern is seen in Europe. The Copenhagen Puberty Study found that the estimated mean age for breast development decreased from 10.9 in 1991 to 9.9 years in 2006, but the average age for menarche didn't change.

It's important to distinguish between a girl who simply starts developing earlier than her friends and a girl with a medical condition. True *precocious* puberty includes girls who have known neuroendocrine disorders or brain tumours (about twenty per cent of cases). These girls may show signs of puberty at ages three or four. In contrast, *early-but-normal* puberty includes healthy girls whose development simply falls to the far left of the bell curve.[75]

True central precocious puberty is relatively rare and has its roots in the brain (the term 'central' meaning central nervous system or brain). In some cases it is caused by the GnRH pulse generator switching on far too early, and if the cause isn't a brain tumour the main treatment involves drugs to block the action of GnRH.

Defining the normal bell curve has been a moving target for the medical community. As you can imagine, continual shifts of what is deemed 'early-but-normal' provoke debate, confusion and misinformation for parents. Girls who start puberty early don't necessarily have a medical problem that needs treatment.

What are the causes of early-but-normal puberty?

Child health has improved considerably since the 1800s. Modern medicine and improved nutrition probably account for some of the shift from menarche occurring in the mid to late teens in the nineteenth century, to around ages eleven or twelve in the girls of the 1960s. However, the current early-but-normal breast development trend of the last couple of decades remains puzzling.

There are numerous theories for the shifting bell curve. The three most well-studied culprits are being overweight, exposure to environmental chemicals that disrupt hormones, and social and psychological stress in early childhood.

Danish studies have concluded that the heavier girls are at age seven, the earlier they enter puberty. Obese children have higher than average levels of a hormone called leptin which stimulates the GnRH in the hypothalamus. But, irrespective of BMI at age seven, there is still a downward trend in the age at which children enter puberty, so obesity isn't the lone culprit.[76]

Endocrine disruptors are chemicals that may interact with or disrupt our hormones. Some are naturally occurring, such as soy, and others are manufactured. One of the most extensively studied chemicals is the plastic Bisphenol A (BPA), once commonly used in baby bottles, but now banned in many countries. The net result of exposure to endocrine disrupters is difficult to predict. But some researchers have commented that they may well be changing girls' hormonal milieu, and in turn how girls' bodies respond to oestrogen.[75]

History supports the 'early childhood stress' theory. Finnish girls evacuated from Helsinki during World War II, girls who survived Hurricane Katrina, and even some of the Project Ice Storm girls entered puberty earlier than expected. While the Christchurch earthquake cohort are still too young to be experiencing puberty, Kathleen Liberty says she will be monitoring those girls over the next few years.

The CATS team found that children who go through early puberty show signs of disruptive behaviour and emotional problems as preschoolers and during their early school years. 'Early puberty may be part of an accelerated transition to adult development which begins early in life. This, in turn, heightens the risks for emotional and behavioural problems,' comments George Patton. He thinks testosterone (for boys) and oestrogens (for girls) might interact with stress-regulation mechanisms from as early as infancy. Patton doesn't scaremonger, and he reminded me that the communities children grow up in can still provide 'social scaffolds' or 'buffers' for early disadvantage. 'Parents remain the most important people in the lives of children, both boys and girls,' he said. 'We can put positive frameworks in place to support these children at this phase of their lives.'

Mood changes at puberty

Girls going through puberty experience frequent, intense and volatile emotions compared to adults and younger children (perhaps toddlers excluded). Tweens seem to experience higher highs and lower lows, and if they do feel happy about something, their positive feelings don't always last as long as in adults. Parents of young girls are probably rolling their eyes at this 'no kidding' statement.

Girls who experience early puberty are more likely to suffer from depression than late bloomers. This doesn't happen to early-developing boys. Instead, boys are more susceptible to depression if they go through puberty *later* than their friends. Interestingly, late-but-normal-developing girls don't show the same risk of depression. In fact, late puberty is protective against depression. It's thought very young girls are poorly equipped emotionally to deal with puberty. There is a mismatch between their maturing bodies and their psychological capacity to cope.

Hormones are the obvious scapegoat for puberty blues. But the rise of oestrogen at puberty cannot take the blame.

In 2015 Australian researchers compiled data from fourteen studies of the effects of oestrogen on mood in adolescent girls. While they found a time-match between rising levels of oestrogen and the emergence of negative moods, there was insufficient data to confirm that oestrogen was the cause. Instead, puberty blues were thought to reflect the adjustment of the brain to the hormonal peaks and troughs of the monthly cycle.[77]

This finding should give us pause for thought. We tend to blame our hormones for emotional instability during pregnancy (baby brain), after giving birth (baby blues) and during menopause (brain fog). But during all these life stages oestrogen is actually neuro-*protective* and *improves* mood.

Finally, don't forget that that puberty in girls involves more than development of a reproductive system capable of producing offspring. Girls also experience:

- ♀ Fine tuning of brain networks.
- ♀ Increased sensitivity of the emotional, social and cognitive brain networks.
- ♀ Shifts in relationships with parents, friends and romantic partners.
- ♀ Shifts in values and morals.
- ♀ The transition from primary school to high school.
- ♀ A growing awareness of the cultural and social expectations of what it means to be a woman, including the realisation that motherhood is a possibility.

The convergence of multiple and challenging physical, cognitive, emotional and social vicissitudes naturally leads to overwhelming feelings. In the words of Hillary Boswell, 'The more we learn about puberty, the less it seems like chaos and more of an incredible metamorphosis that leads to reproductive capacity and psychosocial maturation.' Looking at the list of pubertal experiences, I suggest we should applaud the fact so many girls emerge from puberty emotionally unscathed and thriving!

Normal moods or a mental health problem?

Because puberty is a time renowned for feeling worried, sad or stressed, it's difficult to discern 'normal' moodiness from a mental health problem. Because both boys and girls experience a wide range of emotions and behaviours as part of growing up healthy, any sign in isolation is not necessarily cause for concern. Australia's mental health organisation beyondblue advises that when puberty blues are excessive or prolonged it's important to do more than encourage cosy conversations with parents (which are important), but to also seek professional advice.

All of the experts I spoke to emphasised that attitudes of parents are paramount as to how girls will cope with their changing bodies, regardless of how early, late or average they are. If we don't treat puberty as a crisis or project our own negative experiences onto girls, they'll be much more likely to thrive.

Jocelyn Brewer, a psychologist and school counsellor based in Sydney, Australia, is a strong believer that communication can help solve some of the most tricky problems humans face in relationships. 'Creating rich opportunities for conversation and communicating ideas and sharing experiences is an important way for parents to build connection with kids and have the rapport which might be needed in the teenage years when the need for parental guidance and help seeking is really important,' she says. 'The more young people are nurtured to reflect on experiences and express their ideas, the more of a positive habit it will become.' Learning to deal with negative thoughts and emotions is just as important as learning how to cope with armpit hair or periods.

While writing this chapter, I watched former US First Lady Michelle Obama give her final interview to Oprah Winfrey before leaving the White House. Her words echoed those of many health professionals: 'Children will respond the way they see us respond,' she said. This is as relevant to puberty as it is to politics.

How does puberty shape the brain?

We'll cover in detail what happens in the brain during and after puberty in chapter 5. Up-and-coming neuroscientists take note: most of what we know about the neurobiology of puberty comes from studies of lab animals such as the Syrian hamster and mouse. And we know much more about the role of androgens in the brain than oestrogens. One particular area ripe for research is to uncover how ovarian hormones sculpt the brains and behaviours of teenage girls.

4.

The Menstrual Cycle

ONE OF THE DEFINING MOMENTS OF MY ADOLESCENCE WAS THE arrival of my first period. An avid reader, I'd devoured Judy Blume's *Are You There God? It's Me, Margaret* countless times, and I was desperate for womanhood with its bras, periods and school discos to begin.

My younger sister was the first to hear the news that blood had made its longed-for appearance. I was twelve years and five months old – bang on average. The two of us were on school holidays with our aunty, who laughs remembering how completely unprepared she, a mother of a baby and toddler, was for dealing with her niece's menarche. She had to tear up my baby cousin's cloth nappy into strips to pin into my knickers Judy Blume–style until we made a trip to the tiny local store to stock up on supplies. I was secretly thrilled.

The excitement of menarche out of the way, my period has played little more than a walk-on role in my life since. I've been fortunate to have never suffered serious cramps, heavy bleeding or irregular cycles. In fact, I barely paid attention to its comings and goings until I decided to conceive. Asking around, my nonchalance is clearly not universal. I've heard stories of humiliating dashes to school loos with jumpers tied round blood-stained uniforms, days missed from school or work because of cramps, and problems with infertility and endometriosis.

Our personal monthly neuroscience experiment

Menstruation is one of the few phenomena all biological females experience. Half the world's population spend forty-odd years experiencing monthly fluctuations of hormones and bleeding.

If we look at the menstrual cycle from the perspective of neuroscience, we have a convenient natural experiment for looking at how ovarian hormones influence our brains.

In a typical cycle, oestrogen and progesterone levels oscillate. They're at their lowest in the first few days of bleeding. Oestrogen gradually rises towards the middle of the cycle when ovulation occurs, then drops off again. After ovulation, progesterone dominates then plummets just before bleeding begins.

Because increases in oestrogen precede and then overlap with progesterone, it can be difficult to draw conclusions with regards to the exact role of each hormone, but we can take a good guess. Curious how oestrogen influences mood? Assess mid-cycle emotions. Wonder if falling progesterone impacts memory? Test memory in the days before menstruation.

In this chapter we'll take a look at how monthly cycling of hormones modifies our thoughts and feelings. We'll learn about premenstrual syndrome (PMS) and ask, why do some women suffer from it and others don't? And we'll explore hormonal contraceptives and consider whether you're more likely to be depressed if you're on the pill.

Attitudes to menstruation matter

Let's face it: we're still squeamish talking about periods. Girls are traditionally taught 'menstrual etiquette' whereby periods must be spoken of in strictest privacy, indirectly, and certainly not to boys and men. Lauren Rosewarne, a researcher at the University of Melbourne, has written a book, *Periods in Pop Culture: Menstruation in Film and Television* on how etiquette and attitudes influence women's experiences of their reproductive health.[78]

When I spoke to Rosewarne, she pointed out that despite being a part of everyday life for half the world's population, menstruation is very rarely portrayed on screen or in popular culture. Although part of this is probably because the biologically mundane doesn't make for great TV, Rosewarne believes the problem is when menstruation is portrayed it's as 'a period drama'. 'Periods involve bad moods, floods of blood or social suicide,' she says. 'Because of this I see girls as young as seven feeling anxious about puberty, because they're getting the impression their future periods will be a hassle or a depressing occurrence.' We need to be cautious young girls don't absorb outdated cultural notions about periods being a 'curse' or a source of shame because this can have life-long ramifications.

The neural control of menstruation

Let's get the basic neuroendocrinology lesson out of the way.

As we learned in the previous chapter, levels of FSH, LH, oestrogen and progesterone rise and fall over the menstrual cycle. Their intimate cyclical dance results in ovulation, which neatly divides the month into two phases: the follicular and the luteal phase.

Day one of bleeding marks the start of the follicular phase and is when levels of all ovarian hormones are low. Low levels trigger FSH, which ripens egg-containing ovarian follicles. Over the next week FSH and LH levels climb, stimulating follicles to synthesise oestrogen from cholesterol. As oestrogen levels rise, a positive feedback loop to the brain elicits a large LH surge around day twelve. The LH surge triggers ovulation, typically within twelve to thirty-six hours. Incidentally, LH is the hormone you detect in those over-the-counter ovulation prediction kits. After ovulation, oestrogen manufacture slows and levels then drop sharply towards the end of the luteal phase.

During the follicular phase, progesterone levels remain low, but soar in the days following ovulation when the ruptured follicle (corpus luteum) secretes progesterone. If you take a blood test around day eighteen, you'll find progesterone levels 100-fold greater than oestrogen. Whereas oestrogen builds the endometrial lining of the uterus during the follicular phase, after ovulation progesterone takes over and primes the endometrium for pregnancy.

If the egg is fertilised, it starts to secrete hCG, which ramps up corpus luteum progesterone production until the placenta takes over at around ten weeks' gestation. Rising levels of progesterone feed back to the hypothalamus and pituitary gland inhibiting FSH and LH, and no more eggs mature.

In the absence of a pregnancy and without hCG support, the corpus luteum dies off, progesterone and oestrogen levels plummet, the lining of the uterus stops thickening and bleeding occurs.

This process repeats roughly 450 times through the course of our lives, interrupted only by pregnancies or hormonal contraception, until menopause puts a stop to it altogether.

How do hormones get inside the brain?

'Hormones are peas, and we're all princesses. No matter how many mattresses you put between us and them, hormones still make us squirm,' says Natalie Angier, *New York Times* science journalist, in her book *Woman: An Intimate Geography*.[79] Many of us grew up with this narrative and believe, without question, that hormones control our emotions. We believe we're stuck on an emotional rollercoaster we can't get off.

How, exactly, do hormones influence our emotions?

Oestrogen and progesterone alter the way in which neurons communicate with each other at the synapse, and affect all major neurotransmitter systems including those that use noradrenaline, dopamine, serotonin, glutamate and GABA.

Hormones exert their effects on neurons and other cells by latching on to specific hormone recognition sites called receptors. Hormones can only act on a cell when their receptor is present. Think of a lock and key where the receptor is the lock and the hormone is the key. Turning the key sets off a cascade of biological responses inside the cell.

Receptors for oestrogen are found throughout the brain, mostly in areas associated with reproduction (e.g. the hypothalamus and pituitary), cognition (e.g. the cerebral cortex) and emotion (e.g. the hippocampus and amygdala). Adding another layer of complexity, oestrogen is locally synthesised in the brain, where it may also regulate neural activity. Curiously, there are few human brain studies available for the distribution of progesterone receptors, so we assume from animal studies they're found in broadly the same areas as for oestrogen. The widespread distribution of ovarian hormone receptors and actions on neurons indicates that they have wide-ranging effects on how we think, feel and behave.

One of the most important and well-known effects of oestrogen is on the microstructure of neurons themselves, in particular the dendritic arbour of neurons. Dendrites and spines (tiny buds on dendrites on which synapses form) sprout and retract over the course of the oestrus cycle (the menstrual cycle equivalent in rodents). When levels of oestrogen are highest, spines flourish. When levels of oestrogen drop, spines retract. Our brains are capable of plasticity and the dendritic spine is the major site of this activity. Spines in the hippocampus and cortical areas related to cognition (the fancy neuroscience term for thinking) and emotion regulation are highly sensitive to oestrogen fluctuations.

In humans, we don't have the tools available to look at moment-by-moment effects of oestrogen on neuron microstructure or genes. Instead we must speculate what is happening based on animal work. However, modern neuroimaging techniques such as MRI and fMRI are useful tools to peer into the brains of women to see more broadly how hormones alter brain activity. I like to think of MRI as taking photos of the brain, whereas fMRI takes movies of the brain in action. Both brain-scanning techniques have their flaws, but for now they're the best tools we have.

Imaging the effects of hormones on the brain

A recent systematic review of twenty-four fMRI studies by a group at Uppsala University in Sweden concluded brain activation patterns differ between the follicular and luteal phases of the menstrual cycle or when women take hormonal contraceptives. Brain regions involved in emotion and cognition become more active or less active in response to changing oestrogen or progesterone levels.[80] The review did a good job summarising the 'juvenile' research field; however, the authors were unable to say whether brain activity itself had anything to do with how women actually thought, felt or behaved as their hormone levels went up and down. Lucky for us, two of the authors went on to survey literature that explored exactly this issue.

Does the menstrual cycle change how we feel?

In their paper 'Menstrual cycle influence on cognitive function and emotion processing – from a reproductive perspective', Inger Sundström-Poromaa and Malin Gingnell summarise the findings of eighteen studies exploring how ovarian hormones pacify or provoke emotions.[81]

One set of studies considered how empathy changes across the monthly cycle. Empathy – how able you are to put yourself in someone else's shoes and imagine how they think and feel – is a useful measure of emotional processing. One study showed women photos of faces portraying different emotions (e.g. anger, fear, happiness or disgust) and asked them to name the emotion. Another study had women read short sentences describing real-life situations, such as 'You've lost a precious piece of jewellery' or 'Your child wins a swimming race', and asked them to imagine how they would feel if they were in the same situation.

Results were mixed. Some studies found empathy was lessened – women were less able to recognise and name emotions – during the luteal phase of the cycle, when progesterone levels were high. Other studies found that empathy was unaffected by time of the month.

Another way to measure emotion processing is via tests of emotional memory. Highly emotional events tend to be remembered better than neutral events, a phenomenon we can all attest to. If you've given birth, I doubt you'll ever forget meeting your son or daughter for the first time. And those of us alive in 2001 will have durable memories of the horrific events of 9/11, for example.

Again, results were mixed. Some studies found enhanced memory for emotional items during the luteal phase when progesterone levels are high and oestrogen levels are low, whereas others found no link.

One study robustly linked the luteal phase to traumatic memories. Women were shown highly violent and upsetting film clips and a few days later asked how often scenes from the films had 'spontaneously popped into their minds'. Women consistently reported more intrusive thoughts in the second half of their cycles than the first half.[82]

The tentative conclusion was that the luteal phase and accompanying high levels of progesterone heightened the risk for enhanced emotional memory and perhaps impaired emotion recognition (empathy). But because oestrogen and progesterone work together, and modulate classical neurotransmitters such as serotonin or dopamine, we can't draw a straight line from hormone to brain activity to feelings or actions. I'd also note that this field of research is so new it's practically pre-pubertal. We're not really at the point where we can image a woman's brain, pinpoint her menstrual day and predict from that a thought, mood or behaviour.

Does the menstrual cycle change how we think?

Some people hold very polarised views on sex differences, many centred on cognitive aptitude and women's ability to think and reason. As Margaret McCarthy points out, 'we should never easily accept a scientific conclusion that could be used to justify discrimination or limit opportunities for one sex. No matter how often we repeat that different does not mean better, there is always a tendency to conclude that certain skill sets are superior over others.'[83]

Despite being an archaic notion, the belief that our monthly cycles affect our cognitive skills is widespread. Google it. You'll find headlines such as 'Bleeding On The Job: A Menstruation Investigation. How menstruating at the office can sap women's productivity', or even, 'Periods cripple women's careers', and, of course, Trump's offensive 2016 comment that journalist Megyn Kelly's ability to do her job well was impeded because she 'had blood coming out of her wherever'.

The scientific community has closely investigated these claims by looking at how sex hormones directly alter our capacity to think, reason and remember.

One predominant hypothesis is that we're at our cognitive best at 'masculine' tasks when we're 'least hormonal', and best at 'feminine' tasks when we're 'most hormonal'. Before we go on, I urge you to think back to the introduction when we discussed *d*-values as a measure of the degree of overlap between men's and women's skills.

The best-known example of cognitive sexual dimorphism is mental rotation, which is the ability to rotate 3D objects in your mind. There's plenty of overlap between men's and women's performance, but the average man is better at this than the average woman (even in careful studies it has a *d*-value around 2.0). Reasons given for the gender gap include everything from prenatal testosterone to young boys' proclivity for Lego.[84] One notion is that women excel at 3D rotation only when all hormone levels are low, such as during their periods.

Sundström-Poromaa and Gingnell's reviews found no data supporting this notion. Even when they ditched data from half the studies that had methodological flaws, four of six studies were unable to detect any changes in mental rotation ability due to time of the month.

The Swedes also looked at two classic tests of mental prowess: verbal fluency and verbal memory. Verbal fluency tests ask you to name, say, as many words beginning with the letter 'G' as you can in one minute. Verbal memory tasks involve remembering word lists of random objects such as a shopping list. Verbal fluency and memory also show sexual dimorphism: the average woman performs better than the average man (*d*-values sit around 1.0). It was hypothesised that women should perform better at verbal fluency and memory when oestrogen levels were high. But the review found little evidence in support of this notion either – there were no clear changes in memory ability across the menstrual cycle.

As an aside, I was unable to uncover any decent study on IQ (the best-known measure of intelligence) and the menstrual cycle. There are some people (oddly, none of whom are women) who appear to have a vested interest in proving women's intellectual inferiority. As such they often quote a 2004 meta-analysis[85] that found, on average, men score four to five IQ points higher than women. Numerous subsequent analyses have found no support for this, and critics of the study believed that their methodology was deeply flawed.[86] An example given was that the authors excluded one large study of sex differences in IQ (accounting for forty-five per cent of the total available data). If it had been included, no sex difference would have been found.

This is good news! Our cognitive capabilities and intelligence are not held captive by hormones. We have clear empirical evidence that women can learn, remember and reason during our fertile years and beyond. Who knew?

One of the central tenets of neuroscience and psychology is our ability to thoughtfully regulate our emotions. Our prefrontal cortex (PFC) exerts top-down control over emotion-processing centres such as the amygdala and hippocampus. Learning to identify, understand and manage our emotions isn't just a core life skill we develop during childhood and adolescence: it's a neurobiological reality.

PMS, mood and the menstrual cycle

Clearly, there are only so many deductions we can make about how we think and feel from very granular measures of empathy, verbal memory, 3D mental rotation skills or brain scans. So, let's look more broadly at everyday experiences of mood and the menstrual cycle.

PMS is the collective term for symptoms that show up in the week before your period starts. PMS is widely blamed on low levels of oestrogen combined with the sudden drop in progesterone (if no pregnancy occurs) in the late luteal phase.

Symptoms range from mild to debilitating. Emotional symptoms include mood swings, foggy thinking, anger, tension, weepiness, anxiety, irritability, fatigue, and feeling out of control. Physical symptoms include sore breasts, headaches, migraines, skin problems and bloating. The full list is astonishing and upwards of 150 different symptoms can be used to diagnose PMS.

While writing this book it was extraordinarily difficult to find consensus on how many women actually suffer from PMS. I expected there would be stacks of research and the statistics would be clear-cut. This is not the case.

A Google search reveals PMS affects 'a high percentage of women of childbearing age'. The Women's Health & Research Institute of Australia claims 'most regularly ovulating women' experience some physical and mood symptoms during the premenstrual phase. One meta-analysis found just under half of women globally suffer from PMS; but the prevalence varies across countries. For example, in Iran ninety-five per cent of women claim to suffer from PMS, whereas in France only twelve per cent claim to.[87] To complicate matters, there is also a severe form of PMS called Premenstrual Dysphoric Disorder (PMDD). The literature sets the prevalence of PMDD at somewhere between one per cent and eight per cent.

I can only conclude that somewhere between hardly anyone and almost everyone suffers from PMS.

Is PMS a modern-day myth?

Sarah Romans is a professor of psychological medicine at the University of Otago in New Zealand. Romans runs a clinical psychiatry practice and over the years she's become curious about why women ascribe their irritable moods to PMS. She isn't convinced that the menstrual cycle is the root cause of all mood variability and that women are the 'emotional victims' of their reproductive biology.

In 2012, Romans published a paper in *Gender Medicine* that pooled data from forty-seven studies examining the association between time of the month and mood. Taken together, the studies failed to find any clear evidence of mood changes driven by the phase of the menstrual cycle. In particular, little evidence was found of mood swings or of a specific 'premenstrual negative mood syndrome'.[88]

Subsequent research published in 2013 described how Romans and her team set up the Mood in Daily Life (MiDL) study. They recruited healthy Canadian women between the ages of eighteen and forty-nine and gave them a mobile phone that prompted them with daily questions about mood. Women were asked if they were feeling irritable, on top of things, confident, sad, energetic, weepy and so on. They were also asked about general health and wellbeing, social support, perceived stress and day of menstrual cycle. Tellingly, the women were never told the study was investigating PMS. Over six months 395 menstrual cycles from nearly eighty women were analysed.[89]

The MiDL study found little evidence to support that premenstrual phase by itself influenced mood. Instead, mood was more closely influenced by one of three culprits – lack of social support, perceived stress or poor physical health.

'Knowledge shapes women's own expectations about their health,' says Romans, who told me she uses her research findings daily in the clinic. Romans doesn't believe all women suffer from emotional turmoil before their periods; instead, many women are falsely ascribing their moods to their hormonal status. When she asks her patients to track their daily mood over the course of a few months, only about 'one in twenty' show negative changes in mood that sync with their premenstrual phase. Interestingly, this is a similar proportion of women who are diagnosed with PMDD – the severe clinical form of PMS.

The 'PMS as a myth' concept is one many feminist commentators agree with. 'The notion of premenstrual irrationality, unreliability and irritability is a consistent theme, invariably attributed to raging hormones, and reinforcing the perception of menstruation as a curse,' says Jane Ussher, Professor of Women's Health Psychology, Centre for Health Research, Western Sydney University.[90]

Ussher explains that for millennia, women had their emotions attributed to the 'wandering womb' (the root of the hysteria is derived from the Greek word *hystera*, meaning uterus). The uterus was thought to travel around the body, causing all manner of ailments, with sex and pregnancy the prescribed cure. 'In the Victorian era, the diagnosis of hysteria was widespread, and women's dissatisfaction and marital disobedience were again blamed on the womb,' says Ussher. She points out that even today, cultural images of premenstrual madness abound, with YouTube clips and cartoons depicting the 'premenstrual witch', while self-help books compete to counsel women on coping with PMS.[90]

Romans, Ussher and others believe that negative expectations about PMS have become a self-fulfilling prophecy. 'Many women are diagnosing themselves as having PMDD or PMS and, as a result, not looking for alternative causes for their distress,' says Ussher.[90]

It's worth pointing out the key strength of Romans's research approach. Many studies only ever ask women about their *negative* premenstrual experiences, such as feeling depressed, weepy or irritable. They fail to ask about positive mood, such as feeling happy, energetic or confident. This automatically skews the data towards the negative, and leads to an incomplete and biased description of experiences. 'If only negative mood is studied, it will erroneously be concluded to be the only direction in which mood varies,' says Romans.

Outside of academia, you'd be hard pressed to find a newspaper article or the like talking about women who feel energetic, creative or happy before their periods arrive. There are some 'positive period' movements that encourage women to celebrate and embrace the 'moon time' as a 'sacred goddess' experience. Even if these are empowering concepts for some women, they still generally promote the premenstrual phase as a time for 'nurturing oneself', not necessarily as a time when many women feel upbeat.

Ussher believes premenstrual emotions are an understandable reaction to the stresses and strains of life, and takes the feminist viewpoint that for three weeks of the month women silence their irritation and unhappiness, thus conforming to societal expectations of 'the good woman'. At other times of the month women blame their husbands, workload or lack of sleep for their moods. 'Premenstrually, this self-silencing is broken, but the expression of negative thoughts and feelings is invariably dismissed as PMS,' she says.

Not everyone supports Ussher's and Romans's commentary. Jayashri Kulkarni is one such critic. Kulkarni suggests that the notion PMS is 'all in women's minds as opposed to their endocrinology' ignores the vast body of neuroscience work about the integration of hormones with mental processes.

'Today, we don't have to take the view that women's biology, including their hormone profiles, are unimportant. We can reclaim biology and integrate it with the psychological plus social contexts to see that PMS does exist and does cause real suffering for many women,' she says.[91]

When I spoke to Kulkarni on the phone, she said women may differ in their sensitivity to hormones, perhaps via genetic variations in receptor structure or number. Perhaps women react to hormones similarly to how 'orchid' and 'dandelion' children respond to stress.

Does research dismiss PMS as 'all in your head'? Romans suggests women struggling with this new idea should try to take a more nuanced approach to the causes of their emotions. 'We should consider more broadly what's going on in our lives, and take a look at the quality of our relationships and our physical health before blaming our reproductive function,' she says. I asked Romans how she talks with women who blame their hormones, or who feel their PMS experiences are being dismissed; she said, 'I say to them, "Well, it could be your hormones, let's get some data on that first."' She tries to encourage women to look more broadly at what else is going on in their lives. 'This puzzlingly widespread belief needs challenging, as it perpetuates negative concepts linking female reproduction with negative emotionality,' she says.

Premenstrual Dysmorphic Disorder

PMDD appears to be less controversial, at least among health professionals. It even has its own entry in the psychiatrists' bible, *Diagnostic and Statistical Manual of Mental Disorders* (DSM-5). PMDD is currently considered a type of mood disorder – alongside depression and bipolar disorder. To be diagnosed with PMDD, women must tick five of eleven symptom boxes including: marked mood swings, irritability, anxiety or depression. Symptoms must appear in the week before bleeding, stop once bleeding starts, and be absent the week after bleeding has ended. Symptoms must cause clinically significant distress or interfere with everyday life or relationships. A study in the US found PMDD prevalence sitting at around 1.3 per cent.[92]

There is plenty of debate as to whether PMDD is 'ordinary depression' that gets worse premenstrually, or if it stands alone. DSM-5 is often criticised for 'diagnostic inflation' reducing thresholds for existing disorders, and introduces new disorders resulting in many newly mislabelled 'patients'. In any case, management of PMDD has moved from the gynaecologist's to the psychiatrist's office.

A clue as to the neural origins of PMDD comes from the current best treatment – the antidepressant drug class of selective serotonin reuptake inhibitors (SSRIs). Serotonin is linked to good mood and SSRIs improve mood by increasing the amount of serotonin available in the synapse.

In 2015, Swedish researchers Comasco and Sundström-Poromaa completed a review of the PMDD brain-imaging literature (which, to be honest, is pretty sparse). They found that in women with PMDD the limbic system and PFC aren't working in harmony. Remember that in a healthy adult brain the PFC is able to thoughtfully modulate the emotions emerging from the limbic system. PMDD symptoms might be due to exaggerated 'bottom-up' activity in the limbic brain and blunted 'top-down' activation of the PFC. This type of dysfunctional dialogue between cognition and emotion is commonly seen in depression, and seems to be exacerbated in the luteal phase of women with PMDD.[93]

Does the pill cause depression?

While I was writing this chapter, Romans published another paper with the provocative title 'Crying, oral contraceptive use and the menstrual cycle' using the MiDL study to examine, as the title suggests, the relationship between crying, the pill and time of the month.[94]

'Crying is a mysterious biological and sociocultural phenomenon universally found in human societies with a strongly gendered profile: women cry more than men,' Romans writes. Women in the study reported that they *felt* like crying more often premenstrually and during their period, compared to their mid-cycle phase, but they didn't actually cry more or less at different times of the month. Women on the pill were no more or less likely to cry, or feel like crying compared to naturally cycling women.

There is sparse research on crying itself, but mountains of anecdotes and news headlines claiming the pill makes you sad and weepy, or more prone to everything from weight gain to psychosis. One large study hit global headlines when it was published in *JAMA Psychiatry* in September 2016.[95] 'It's not in your head: Striking new study links pill to depression' announced newspaper headlines. 'We knew it! You're finally taking us seriously,' replied women around the globe.

The study, which was conducted in Denmark, accessed fourteen years' worth of health data from more than one million Danish women aged fifteen to thirty-four. The researchers asked the simple question: Is use of hormonal contraception associated with treatment of depression?

Danish health data tracked which women took hormonal contraception (over half the women in the study) including varied contraceptive methods (combined pill, implants and intrauterine devices – IUDs), and data also indicated who was diagnosed with depression. A depression diagnosis was counted if women were given an antidepressant prescription (thirteen per cent of all women in the study), or diagnosed with depression in a psychiatric hospital (two per cent of all women in the study).

The study concluded that use of hormonal contraceptives, especially among adolescents, was indeed associated with subsequent use of antidepressants and a first diagnosis of depression. But before you throw out your pill packet, let's take a closer look at the results.

For all women in the study, there was a twenty-three per cent increase in *relative risk* of being prescribed antidepressants after beginning the pill. Data revealed that the outcome was worse for teens, with an eighty per cent increased *relative risk* of developing depression on the pill. Newspapers widely reported this finding. But some headlines got it very wrong and stated that eighty per cent of all women on the pill get depressed.

It is really important to understand how 'risk' gets reported. Relative risk (which was reported in the newspapers) is one of two ways to describe the same statistic. Relative risk tells us very little, but it sounds impressive and often scary. *Absolute risk*, on the other hand, tells you how likely it is that the something will actually happen to you.

Looking at the data from an absolute risk perspective we see 2.1 per cent of women taking the pill filled a script for antidepressants, compared to 1.7 per cent of women not on the pill. Or in simpler terms, take 100 women and over the course of a year, *less than one extra woman* on the pill will be prescribed an antidepressant.

For all the women taking the pill, 0.30 per cent were admitted to a psychiatric hospital; by comparison, for all women *not* taking the pill, 0.28 per cent were admitted to a psychiatric hospital (we can assume women admitted to hospital had serious cases of depression). The absolute risk for psychiatric admission when on the pill was tiny.

The Royal College of Obstetricians and Gynaecologists in the UK states that based on the Danish data, an honest doctor would simply have to tell her patient that, on average, only one in 221 women exposed to hormonal contraception over a year is likely to subsequently be prescribed an antidepressant. And only one in 2441 women is likely to be diagnosed with depression at a psychiatric hospital.[96]

The statistics simply do not support headlines that state the pill *causes* depression in eighty per cent of women.

What was rarely reported was the finding that after taking hormonal contraceptives for a year, the (small) increased risk for depression in teenagers wore off. And it's entirely possible the younger women were more susceptible because teens are more vulnerable to developing depression anyway.

There is a big 'but' to the soothing advice issued by the Royal College: not everyone with depression takes antidepressants, and not everyone seeks help if they're feeling blue.

What happens to your brain on the pill?

For many women, even a modest reduction in general wellbeing when taking the pill is not worth the contraceptive benefit. Many of us have probably experienced mood swings, irritability or other emotional issues when we're on the pill – symptoms that aren't severe enough to warrant an antidepressant prescription or psychiatric admission. This may explain the high discontinuation rate and irregular use of the pill as a contraceptive method.

In 2017, a study published in the journal *Fertility and Sterility* found that healthy women reported reduced quality of life, mood and physical wellbeing after taking a common birth control pill for three months.

The study from the Karolinska Institutet was a double-blind, randomised, placebo-controlled trial which meant that neither the researchers giving out the pills nor the women taking them knew whether they were getting a placebo (sugar pill) or contraceptive pill. All 340 healthy women (aged eighteen to thirty-five) filled out surveys on wellbeing and mental health at the beginning and end of the study. The women on the pill rated their quality of life to be significantly lower during the study than those who were given placebos. Both general quality of life and specific aspects like mood, wellbeing, self-control, vitality and energy level were affected negatively by the contraceptives. Unlike the Danish million-women study, no significant increase in depression was observed.[97]

Sometimes alternative methods of contraception fix symptoms. I can personally attest to this scenario when I felt one version of the combined pill left me feeling emotionally out of control (precisely one of the outcomes of the Karolinska study). On the recommendation of an insightful women's health nurse I switched pill brands and never looked back.

When weighing up pros and cons of depression or wellbeing versus the pill, we need to carefully consider why we might want to use hormonal contraception. Not only does the pill have many positive health benefits such as reducing cancer risk, avoiding pregnancy is hardly a trivial health outcome. Hormonal contraceptives are among the most reliable forms of birth control, and can be a great way to reduce anxiety around the potential of an unplanned pregnancy.[98] As we'll explore in later chapters, pregnancy and childbirth can make you pretty blue too.

One possible mechanism whereby the pill may affect general wellbeing is a direct negative effect of the progestin (synthetic progesterone) component in the pill on the brain. Progesterone can exert a sedative effect on the brain, and dampens down neural activity. 'Although we did not find statistically significant effects on depressive symptoms,' say the authors of the Karolinska Institutet study, 'it is possible that a direct progestin-induced central nervous system effect could be the underlying mechanism behind reduced wellbeing, self-control and vitality in the oral contraceptive group.'[97]

Different hormonal contraceptives work in different ways. For example, the combined oestrogen/progestin contraceptive formula inhibits release of GnRH, and in turn LH and FSH, thus preventing ovulation (see how that earlier endocrine lesson is coming in handy!). Progesterone-only pills work in roughly the same way. Progesterone-only IUDs don't prevent ovulation; instead they make the uterus more hostile for both sperm and eggs if they are released.

The implications of the pill are complex because it both suppresses your natural levels of ovarian hormones and simultaneously elevates levels of synthetic hormones for very short bursts every day (the half-life of synthetic hormones is only a few hours, which is why you need to take the pill daily).

We surmise that synthetic hormones cause the same changes to brain structure and neurochemistry as natural hormones do, in the short term at least. These changes probably underlie the reported increased risk of depression and mood changes – both good and bad. But believe it or not, no-one has yet looked at the long-term effects of the pill on the brain.

As with the menstrual cycle, most studies of the pill have looked at sexually dimorphic behaviours (i.e. those that differ between males and females). Not that men take the pill, of course, but the assumption is that these behaviours may be under the influence of ovarian hormones.

In terms of tests of cognitive ability (3D mental rotation, verbal fluency and memory), the results are mixed. Some studies report better mental rotation performance in pill users – so women on the pill perform more like many men. Other studies show enhanced verbal memory when on the pill – some women on the pill perform more like, well, women.

Reports on mood are equally inconsistent. Some women report feeling more emotionally stable on birth control (especially if they experiment with finding a pill that works for them) but others report depression, anxiety, fatigue, neurotic symptoms, compulsion and anger. It's like there are two populations of women with differential emotional responses to sex hormones. Jayashri Kulkarni's orchid–dandelion hypothesis might yet prove to be correct.

A 2014 overview of this field can be found in the open access journal *Frontiers in Neuroscience*, published with the alluring title: '50 years of hormonal contraception – time to find out what it does to our brain'. Sadly, it's not yet time to find out that much: the authors say they could only summarise 'sparse findings'.[99]

Clearly, this is yet another pre-pubertal field of study, and despite more than fifty years of oral contraceptive use by millions of women around the globe, all researchers can conclude is that 'there is a strong demand for additional studies'.

With all the talk about suppressing ovulation, let's not forget, our brains use hormones and emotions to drive us towards lust, love, sex, pleasure and procreation (not simply towards irritability, depression and anxiety!).

5.

The Teenage Brain

A FEW YEARS AGO, MY HUSBAND AND I CELEBRATED OUR JOINT fortieth birthdays with a 1990s-themed party. I wore a blue Monica Lewinsky–style dress, one friend came as *Pulp Fiction*'s Mia Wallace, and there were plenty of double-denim ensembles, Doc Martens and pirate shirts. Our playlist was dominated by the music of Oasis, Blur, Coldplay and U2. Despite growing up on opposite sides of the world, in New Zealand and Ireland, my husband and I have found that very similar soundtracks accompanied the memories of our teens and early twenties – songs our boys now hilariously call 'Dad music'.

Nostalgia for the music you loved in your teens is commonplace and can teach us a lot about the heightened plasticity of adolescent social, emotional and cognitive brain networks.

The songs from your halcyon days feel like 'your music' because music choice has important social consequences when you're young. As teens we're strongly driven to find a new tribe. Part of the desire to fit in means teens are exquisitely sensitive to being left out. Teens just want to be accepted and valued members of a tribe, so they'll do their best to dress alike, share interests and listen to the same music.

Passions run deep during adolescence. Emotions add colour and resonance to our lives and also send the signal, 'Hey, this is what's important.' We have a strong tendency to remember events (good and bad) that have an emotional component because the brain pays attention to and 'tags' such memories as important.

Many adults have what is called a 'reminiscence bump', or particularly vivid memories of the thrilling years between ten and thirty. Compared with our childhood or midlife, we have superior recall of the books we read, films we watched, parties we attended and the accompanying soundtracks.

Adolescence is proving to be a phase of heightened brain plasticity – your capacity to learn peaks and the memories forged are particularly indelible. However, with enhanced plasticity comes increased vulnerability. As Natalie Angier says, 'Who can forget adolescence? And who has ever recovered from it?'[79]

Halfway between girlhood and womanhood

Biology determines the beginning of adolescence. The *tick-tick-tick* of the hypothalamic clock signals the beginning of the transition from girl to woman. The end of adolescence has no clear biological demarcation. When exactly do girls become adults? When they're physically able to have a baby? Or when they actually have a baby? When they turn eighteen? Finish school? Leave home? Get their first full-time job? Buy a house? Get married? With puberty starting earlier than it used to and the traditional cultural markers of adulthood somewhat irrelevant, 'adolescence' could last decades! Because adolescence mostly spans the teenage years, in this chapter I'll use the two terms interchangeably.

Despite its current unclear cultural or social endpoint, biologically adolescence is a distinct period of brain development. It's when the brain becomes particularly vulnerable to reorganisation by sex hormones and when the cognitive, emotional and social circuits refine and mature. Tracking alongside the brain changes are the stereotypical changes to the thoughts, emotions and behaviours of the brain's teenage owner.

The stereotype of the teenage brain is wrong

Let's be honest, we have a tendency to wring our hands over all the things that can go wrong for girls in their teenage years. We hope like heck our daughters emerge as healthy well-rounded women who've avoided pregnancy, eating disorders, depression, bullying, sexual assault, drugs and the modern-day pitfalls of social media addiction and online harassment.

As well as being schooled on how to avoid all of the above, teenage girls have to contend with neuroscience explanations as to why their 'immature' brains make them so vulnerable to such vices. The assumption seems to be that the teenage years are a minefield and many girls are unlikely to survive unscathed.

A few years ago, researchers in the UK took the unusually insightful step of asking a group of eighty-five teenagers what their thoughts were on neuroscience explanations of 'the teenage brain'. Intriguingly, most participants weren't that interested in what neuroscience could teach them about themselves. Some said it was 'boring', whereas others found it intrusive and unseemly, turning teenagers into 'oddities', alienating them, underscoring their relative powerlessness and threatening their agency. (If you're a neuroscientist, I'm sorry, they don't seem to care much for your work.) 'Do we want to see into adult brains? So why teenage brains?' asked one.

The young people who took part in the survey were smart enough to see the potential for neuroscience research, but felt it could be better used to obtain insights into teen behaviour without using it to pile on the usual load of moral judgement and stereotyping. 'Teenagers are often misunderstood, and it might be helpful if people knew how they think, see their point of view,' was one response, and, 'It will help defeat stereotypes,' said another.[100]

Adults seem to find both humour and horror in the concept of the adolescent brain. Somehow, we forget about the many positive outcomes that result from owning and operating such adaptable neural circuitry. Young women can be wonderfully compassionate, empathic and devoted friends, passionate advocates for causes they believe in, highly motivated and goal-oriented, and they're at the peak of their learning potential and creativity.

So, on behalf of teenage girls everywhere, let us begin a careful and objective exploration of their brains.

The teenage brain is still undergoing development

Most scholars agree on three facts about the teenage brain.[101]

First, brain structure continues to change between childhood and adulthood. Grey matter volume peaks at puberty, then declines throughout adolescence and into the twenties. White matter volume increases throughout childhood, adolescence and into adulthood.

Second, girls' brains mature slightly faster than boys'. This sex difference in brain development is in sync with physical development where, on average, girls enter puberty a year or two before boys, who then quickly catch up.

Third, different brain regions mature at different rates. Development of the limbic system, which drives emotions, speeds up at puberty, but the PFC, which is involved in thinking and judgement, doesn't mature until our twenties. This causes a 'developmental mismatch' between emotion and reward processing, and thinking and judgement. The mismatch determines aspects of teenage behaviour such as being overly emotional, impulsive and hypersensitive to social situations.

Grey matter thins as connections are refined

The prefrontal cortex, as its name suggests, sits at the front of the brain and is sometimes called the brain's CEO because it acts as a wise leader, exerting top-down control over other brain areas. The PFC is involved in emotion regulation, judgement, strategy, impulse control, attention, working memory and social cognition – navigating complex social relationships such as discerning friend from 'frenemy' from foe.

During childhood, the grey matter of the PFC continues to thicken as neurons make new synapses, much like a tree growing extra branches, twigs and roots. During the teens, thinning occurs across much of the cortex but is most obvious in the PFC.

Loss or thinning of grey matter always sounds unhealthy, but as is often the case with the brain, less is more. Grey matter loss is vitally important and is due to pruning away of unwanted 'twigs and branches', which partly depends on experience in a 'use it or lose it' manner. Connections that are being used are strengthened and those that aren't being used are pruned away.

More white matter enables faster communication

MRI scans have revealed ever-increasing volumes of white matter in the tracts leading to and from the PFC during adolescence. Recall that axons are insulated by myelin, which speeds up signalling between brain regions. Myelinated axons transmit impulses up to 100 times faster than unmyelinated axons, and faster transmission means faster mental processing.

Jay Giedd, a neuroscientist at the University of California, San Diego, has found that increased white matter means the connections between brain regions become stronger and more numerous. The brain matures by becoming more interconnected and more specialised.

To use Giedd's metaphor, brain maturation is not so much a matter of adding new letters to the alphabet but one of combining existing letters into words, words into sentences and sentences into paragraphs. 'These changes ultimately help the brain to specialise in everything from complex thinking to being socially adept,' he says.[102]

Subcortical brain areas shrink and grow

Changes to white and grey matter structure are not restricted to the PFC. Subcortical brain structures start to mature right around puberty, and development is more or less complete by the mid-teenage years.

Subcortical brain regions are those deep inside the brain under ('sub') the cortex in the frontal and temporal lobes. They include the limbic system (hippocampus and amygdala), and the corpus striatum, which is made up of four parts: nucleus accumbens, caudate, putamen and globus pallidus. They're connected to the PFC and to each other by bundles of axons.

In girls, the amygdala and hippocampus get bigger during puberty. At the same time, the four structures making up the corpus striatum all shrink. Maturation of subcortical structures is fastest in late childhood and early adolescence but the rate of growth or shrinkage slows right down after age sixteen.[103, 104]

The social brain develops during adolescence

The 'social brain' includes brain areas involved in social cognition – skills allowing us to navigate the complexities of relationships, attract a mate, discern friend from foe, and recognise the thoughts and feelings of others. Social brain networks include the PFC, cortical regions involved in face processing, and also a specific region called the temporoparietal junction (TPJ). The TPJ is situated where the temporal and parietal lobes meet. If you scratch your head just above and back a bit from your ear, you'll be in about the right spot.

During adolescence, the social brain architecture refines and adult-like patterns of neural activity emerge. Maturation of social behaviours tracks alongside the changes in brain structure and activity.

Teenage brains join a new tribe

During childhood, girls have their most intimate relationships with their parents and siblings, explains psychologist Lisa Damour in her fascinating book *Untangled: Guiding Teenage Girls Through the Seven Transitions into Adulthood*. 'Girls break up with their parents when they become teenagers,' she says.[105] As girls mature, they aren't just looking to make new friends; part of the process of growing up is replacing family with a tribe that they can feel proud to call their own.

Because belonging to a new tribe is so critically important to girls, being at odds with or different from their friends leads to distress. Damour says she can't overstate the significance of a teenager's tribe membership, 'The fear of being tribeless – distanced from one's family yet without a peer group – cuts to the quick and leads to the idealisation of popularity and the social connections that come with it.'[105]

There is a strong evolutionary drive to leave the family nest and explore. All young social animals, from puppies to porpoises, would rather frolic with their friends than their parents. 'Social reorientation' or the shift of focus from self and family to same-age friends is deeply biological – it diminishes the likelihood of inbreeding and creates a healthier genetic population.

The painful consequences of being left out

If you're feeling brave, cast your mind back to your teenage years and recall a time when you felt excluded. Most of us won't have to think too hard to remember a time (real or imagined) we weren't invited to a party or trip to the mall or sleepover. Remember those dreadful popularity-ranking lists that were penned and passed around the class? For those of us who fell near the bottom of the list, weren't invited to the party or were the target of taunting (and that was all of us at one time or another), it was exquisitely painful. Girls have a particular knack for meanness and passive–aggressive bullying such as freezing someone out, spreading cruel gossip or deliberate exclusion, and meanness and bullying are a big cause of sadness, depression and self-harm in teenage girls.[106]

The fear of being left out or ostracised threatens some of our most fundamental human needs, such as self-esteem, feeling like a valued member of a group and our sense of meaningful existence. Cruel as it sounds, researchers can deliberately induce the feelings of exclusion in order to study them.

In one such game called Cyberball, invented by Purdue University psychologist Professor Kipling Williams, participants play online catch with two other 'players'. After a few throws of the virtual ball, the other 'players' stop throwing the ball to the participant, who has been led to believe they're playing with real people, but it's actually a pre-programmed computer game. They're also told that a skill such as mental visualisation is being assessed (telling them they're about to be manipulated into feeling left out kind of defeats the purpose). Many thousands of young people and adults have played Cyberball and it reliably induces feelings of rejection, anger and sadness in the ostracised player even if they play for only a few minutes.

'Being excluded or ostracised is an invisible form of bullying that doesn't leave bruises, and therefore we often underestimate its impact,' says Williams. He says that being left out, whether it's by friends or strangers, can be excruciating. And the painful feelings last for a long time.[107]

Professor Sarah-Jayne Blakemore is a University College London neuroscientist, credited with creating the discipline of adolescent brain development and for showing adolescence as a time of remarkable plasticity and sensitivity to social and educational experiences.

Using fMRI, Blakemore has compared social brain responses to rejection in teenage girls and adult women. In one Cyberball study of nineteen girls (aged fourteen to sixteen) and sixteen adult women, the girls found social exclusion far more upsetting than the adults. The teenagers' inability to regulate their distress played out in their brains. In a social brain area known to regulate negative feelings – the left ventrolateral PFC – neural activity was lower in teens than adults. Blakemore suggests 'increased sensitivity to rejection in adolescence may result from reduced regulation of social distress'.[108]

Teen brains are primed to like the same things as their friends, including music. In a paper called 'Neural Mechanisms of the Influence of Popularity on Adolescent Ratings of Music', a team from Emory University describes how they used fMRI to scan the brains of thirty-two twelve- to seventeen-year-olds while they listened to music and rated how much they liked each song. The first time the teens listened, they had no idea of the popularity of the song, but the second time around they were told a song's ranking, and given the opportunity to change their own rating if they wanted to. As you might expect, teenagers were strongly influenced by a song's popularity. Tellingly, they often altered their rating of a song after they were told how popular it was, to align their choice with others'.

The fMRI scans revealed brain regions associated with anxiety and negative emotions were activated when the teens realised the music they liked was unpopular, what the authors call 'mismatch anxiety'. Part of what drives a teenager's need to 'fit in' is the social anxiety they feel when they're left out. When the teens changed their ratings to match and 'fit in' with their peers, their anxiety dissipated.[109]

Why does rejection hurt so badly?

When we feel rejected or left out, we use words like 'hurt feelings', 'broken heart' or 'kicked in the guts'. And the loss of someone we love is almost certainly one of the most crushingly painful of life's experiences. Why are negative social experiences so 'painful'?

One theory proposes that this is because physical pain and social pain share similar neural networks. It makes sense that threats to social connection or feeling excluded utilise the same pain signal that signifies threat to the physical body. Fitting in with a tribe is akin to survival. This theory finds support from fMRI studies and observations that the experience of physical pain can be lessened in the presence of social support.[110]

The notion that the two types of pain are neurologically similar has led to some unusual ideas about how to treat social pain, including using traditional painkillers. Opiates, best known for their pain-relieving effects, reduce separation anxiety in baby lab rats. And paracetamol alleviates social anxiety and feelings of rejection when playing Cyberball.[111]

The idea that painkillers are 'emotion relievers' has started to catch on. Many health professionals are understandably alarmed. The NHS in the UK has gone so far as to release a statement saying, 'Don't take paracetamol for painful emotions.' And it should go without saying, the studies I've described here are not a green light for taking paracetamol or opiates to 'treat' feelings of loneliness, distress or emotional pain.

The 'emotional adolescent' is developmentally normal

Teenage girls are very emotional creatures. But not all teenage girls experience 'storm and stress'. When I was seventeen, my levels of anxiety during final-year high-school exams were so out of control I ended up at the family GP being treated for panic attacks. But the vast majority of my teen years were joyful, empowering and a whole lot of fun.

Sarah Whittle is an associate professor of psychiatry at the University of Melbourne, where she specialises in adolescent brain development and resilience. Whittle explained to me that the emotional lives of teenage girls differ from adults because of the 'developmental mismatch' between their 'rational PFC' and 'emotional limbic brain'. 'It's still only a theory,' she reminds me, 'but the evidence is stacking up that hyperactivity of the limbic system is responsible for heightened emotional reactivity in adolescents. As the PFC matures, its ability to regulate the activity in subcortical structures improves.'

Learning to regulate emotions

Being able to calmly assess and keep emotions in check is a crucial life skill. Emotional regulation lets us navigate changing social landscapes and foster mental wellbeing. One of the most effective ways to regulate your emotions is a technique called cognitive reappraisal. Cognitive reappraisal changes the way you interpret a situation, which in turn calms your hot-headed response.

Imagine you're fourteen and walking up to the front door of a party. Inside you can hear all your girlfriends laughing hysterically. Your appraisal of the situation might be, 'OMG! They're laughing about me behind my back.' That appraisal (correct or not) will likely trigger intense feelings of sadness and rejection, and might quickly be followed by the thought, 'They hate me. I'm going home!'

A different way of thinking about the situation – the reappraisal – might be, 'Sure, they're laughing. Perhaps someone told a funny joke. Maybe I should go inside and find out.' The reappraisal (correct or not) encourages you to consider different perspectives, and leads to a way of thinking that keeps a lid on emotional distress. Adults are much better at cognitive reappraisal than children and teens. We're more experienced with a range of social situations and better at deploying the thinking skills required.

The neural basis of cognitive reappraisal is studied by eliciting negative emotions with provocative or distressing photos comprised of images that range from neutral (furniture or landscapes) to horrific or exciting scenes (mutilated bodies or erotic nudes). Whittle's research shows that teenage girls find the photos much more emotionally disturbing or arousing than adults. In her lab, fMRI shows that deploying the skill of cognitive reappraisal activates a distributed cortical network including the PFC, which in turn down-regulates excitability in the limbic system.

Emotional regulation skills don't always magically appear as we mature, but they can be formally taught. Whittle coaches her teenage volunteers in cognitive reappraisal by encouraging them to think, 'This isn't real, it's a scene from a movie', or, 'The situation looks worse than it is', or, 'It could be a lot worse', or, 'At least it is not me in that situation'.[112]

Is mental illness emotional development gone wrong?

One theme in adolescent brain research can be summed up by the phrase 'moving parts get broken'. Because the teenage brain is undergoing such extensive remodelling, it's thought that it's easy for the wiring to go awry, predisposing girls to depression, anxiety and eating disorders. The emotional life of teenage girls is complex both inside and out. It's clear that 'inside' hormones are fluctuating and neural networks are fine-tuning. But we tend to forget the dynamic shifts taking place 'outside'.

Many emotions girls experience are novel, especially those taking place in new social contexts. There is a first time for everything and that includes your first crush (especially if it's unrequited), experience of jealousy, being left off the party invite list, and getting likes on Instagram. The newness of these experiences heightens their emotional impact. Sometimes this is positive – falling in love for the first time is pretty wonderful! Sometimes this is negative – being rejected by your first love is rather painful.[113]

Girls' preference for emotional intimacy increases during their early teenage years and intense 'bosom buddy' friendships form around the same time girls 'break up' with their families. This leaves girls potentially vulnerable if those friendships break down or are less than ideal. Loss of friendship is a significant and overlooked potential cause of stress.

While the 'wrong' friendships can lead teens astray, the 'right' kinds of friends are powerful and protective. I had one such dear friend all through high school (we're still close now and I've called on her psychiatric training to inform sections of this book). While writing this chapter we talked about how our devoted friendship buffered us from the tumult so many of our peers experienced. We know the happiest teens aren't the ones who have the most 'friends' on Instagram but the ones who have a few close supportive friendships, and sometimes that means having one terrific friend.

Risk-taking and the mismatch between thinking and feeling

One prevailing view is that because the brain is 'undergoing renovation' the impulsive teenager is more likely to engage in risky behaviours. They crash cars (if they're boys) or get pregnant (if they're girls). Rightfully so, critics argue that this view is somewhat over-generalised and focuses on teenagers as 'deviant risk-takers'.

Sure, teenagers *are* more inclined towards risky behaviours than adults or children, but social adventure, sensation seeking and even blue hair and half-naked selfies are not signs of delinquency. They're a normal part of testing out new tribes and trying on new identities for size.

It's also worth pointing out that not all young people make 'bad' decisions, and not all risky behaviour leads to a negative outcome; what might seem tame to one person might be perceived as highly reckless to another. The most deviant act I got up to during high school (I'm now less horrified at myself than I was at the time) was helping a friend break into a classroom one weekend. She levered open a window, I hoisted her in and then stood guard. She'd forgotten her homework folder and didn't want to turn up on Monday without it complete. Clearly, the prospect of unfinished homework was more threatening to us than the risk of being caught breaking and entering the school.

Do girls take risks?

The statistics are clear when it comes to male versus female harmful risk-taking. The Dunedin Study has found that boys and men disproportionately outnumber girls and women in risky behaviours such as using drugs, vandalism and theft.[114] Young men are more likely than young women to die in car accidents as a result of dangerous driving. And boys and men are more likely to participate in adventure sports or win a Darwin Award – the posthumous award given annually to a person who has died doing something stupendously stupid.

A 1999 meta-analysis of gender and risky behaviour found that males tend to take risks even when a risk is obviously a *bad* idea.[115] The same analysis found the opposite was true for girls and women – we're less likely to take risks even in a fairly innocuous situation, including when it might even be a *good* idea to do so, such as intellectual risk-taking in exams or entrepreneurship. Sheryl Sandberg, COO of Facebook, has made famous the finding that men apply for a job when they meet only 60 per cent of the qualifications, but women apply only if they meet 100 per cent. Because of this difference (again, average differences, plenty of overlap), men and boys tend to encounter more failure and, sadly, girls and women tend to experience less success. Sandberg is on to something.

There are many social and cultural reasons for the differing propensity for risk, but the most popular theory is that the testosterone makes men risk-takers, and lack of testosterone makes women risk-avoiders. By this point in the book you should automatically question such a simplistic 'bottom-up biology trumps all' notion. The data certainly don't support it. Testosterone levels rarely predict a propensity for risk in a neat join-the-dots way. Curiously high *and* low levels of testosterone are correlated with risk aversion in men *and* women (remember that the ovaries and female adrenal glands trickle out testosterone). As Cordelia Fine says, 'rather than being a king who issues orders', testosterone is just another voice in the crowd.[116]

The imaginary audience – who is watching me?

Part of being a successful tribe member and learning to be a good friend is developing the ability to read the emotions of others. Social emotions – such as guilt, embarrassment, shame and pride – require the specific ability to recognise someone else's state of mind. That is, appreciating that someone else thinks and feels in a way different from yourself.

We start to develop 'theory of mind', as it's called, as very young children. The process of mentalising is even more sophisticated. It involves recognising the needs, desires, feelings, beliefs and reasons of others. Mentalising is one of the most complex tasks humans have to master. We see mastery emerge clearly in the behaviour of teenage girls as they become super-sensitive and worried about what others think about them.

This can be positive. Many teenage girls are passionate adopters of social causes and volunteerism. But the increased awareness of the minds of others at the same time as shifting away from the security of childhood provides a perfect storm for 'the imaginary audience'. It's worth noting that adolescent egocentrism is a normal part of development, but due to the pervasiveness of social media, girls are even more sensitive to what others think than those of us from older generations. The 'imaginary audience' is a whole lot bigger and less imaginary than it was even a decade ago.[117]

'It seemed like such a good idea at the time' is a common excuse and reflects the simple fact that teenagers often make bad decisions because the potential feel-good reward outweighs the bad. What we've learned from research is that risky behaviour is driven more by pleasure than by pain. Decision-making and risk-evaluation don't happen in isolation. Both the emotional brain (feelings of reward and pleasure) and the social brain (peer influence) are involved. The reward is clear: tribe approval.

A classic study published in the journal *Developmental Psychology* in 2005 was designed to measure whether teens really are more easily swayed to take risks in the presence of an audience.

Researchers recruited 306 volunteers from three age groups: young teens (thirteen to sixteen), young adults (eighteen to twenty-two) and adults (twenty-four and older). Each volunteer was asked to bring along two close friends to watch them complete the challenge – a simulated driving game called Chicken. Chicken measures in-the-moment risk-taking and drivers are rewarded based on how quickly they finish driving their car through a virtual town. For example, at some intersections the subjects are faced with a decision: brake for the orange light or speed up (chance a crash) but complete the game faster.

As you might expect, the youngest teens took significantly more risks than the adults when their friends were watching them play. But here's what was surprising: when they were driving 'alone' they took the *same* number of driving risks as older teens or adults.

Clearly, young teenagers are perfectly capable of evaluating danger and making smart decisions – they can do it when they're alone. They just seem to lose their minds in 'hot' situations. 'Hot cognition' is a hypothesis that recognises that our thinking is influenced by our emotional state. Peer pressure or having an imaginary audience (your mum might have called it showing off) switches teens into 'hot cognition' mode.[118]

We all know that getting up to mischief with your friends is much more fun than going it alone. Tellingly, an fMRI version of the Chicken driving game found that the ventral striatum in the brain involved in motivation, pleasure and anticipation of reward was more strongly activated in teenagers when they were driving with friends versus driving alone. In teenagers subcortical dopamine pathways mature before the rational 'why don't you think it over' PFC does.

In the case of teenagers, driving too fast in cars gains approval of the tribe. For some teenage girls (myself included), peer approval might not come from driving fast. For me and my friends, getting homework in on time was the priority! Social context matters. Choose your friends wisely.

Adolescence is a unique window of opportunity for education

As we've seen, risk-taking is typically framed as undesirable. But at school taking a risk can be useful. 'The adolescent brain is malleable and adaptable – this is an excellent opportunity for learning and creativity,' writes Blakemore.[119] Taking a risk by asking a question in class or providing an answer that goes beyond the information in the textbooks is a vital skill that enables progress.

Giedd agrees the new insights of adolescent neuroscience will encourage adolescents to challenge their brain with the kinds of skills that they want to excel at for the remainder of their lives. 'They have a marvellous opportunity to craft their own identity and to optimise their brain,' he writes.[102] An adolescent's success in pursuing long-term academic, athletic or artistic goals, for example, typically requires motivation to practise the relevant skills and a desire to persevere through difficulties. Their brains are primed for success.

It's a rather lovely coincidence of modern life that girls are attending high school at the peak of their learning potential. The regions of the brain that are plastic and undergoing refinement are the exact same regions involved in skills related to selective attention, reasoning, logic and memory. Take learning mathematics. Moving from understanding basic arithmetic to the symbolic language of algebra, generalising, modelling and analysing equations needs abstract reasoning skills, logic, mental imagery and creative thinking. These are precisely the skills the teen brain is mastering and refining.

Blakemore has commented that adolescence represents a period of brain development during which environmental experiences are crucial. 'If early childhood is seen as a major opportunity or a sensitive period for teaching, so too might adolescence.'[119]

The teenage years are a unique stage of enhanced plasticity and adaptability for the brain. 'With increased opportunity comes increased vulnerability,' Professor George Patton said to me. 'Vulnerability goes hand in glove with opportunity.' I, like many other researchers in the field, feel we should focus on the teenage years not as a time of storm and stress but of unparalleled opportunity for learning and creativity.

6.

Depression and Anxiety

MY FIRST MINOR BRUSH WITH ANXIETY WAS AT AGE TEN WHEN I found myself in a perfect storm: the onset of puberty, a bout of glandular fever and a grandparent with cancer. This culminated in what I've since self-diagnosed as childhood separation anxiety. My memories of 1985 aren't so much of the sore throats, fatigue and weeks off school – rather, they're fits of extreme anxiety based on the utter conviction that someone in my family was going to die.

I'd spend the hours and even days in advance of Mum leaving the house in a state of cold prickling fear. Part of my disordered response when she did go out was to set off on little solo search parties. I remember two occasions when I climbed out a window in my pyjamas, and once walked out of school, ostensibly to save her from dying.

My 'fretting', as we called it, was never dismissed, but being the mid-80s it wasn't treated either. Today I might have visited a child psychologist for cognitive behavioural therapy or counselling. But as it happened, like many childhood difficulties, I eventually grew out of it.

I experienced a second brush with anxiety at age seventeen. It wasn't serious or long-lasting but the timing couldn't have been worse. My susceptibility to anxiety (separation disorder increases the risk of panic disorders during young adulthood) met with my belief that life began and ended with final-year high-school exams.[120]

For the most part, my preparation went well. But the afternoon before my biology final I was sitting at my desk studying when I was overcome with a sense of impending doom, and cold fear that prickled up and down my spine. I felt oddly detached – I knew I was safe and I'd long grown out of worrying about Mum, but it was all very overwhelming. I started crying and couldn't stop. With Mum's help we threw everything we had at it: I closed the books, took a long walk, had a nice meal and a good night's sleep, but when I sat down in the exam hall the next morning, the doom and fear slammed into me again and I ran from the hall. When Mum took me to our lovely GP, he expressed genuine surprise. He'd never before seen exam-related anxiety in a teenage girl.

Twenty-five years later, and a survey of 722 Year 12 students from a range of schools in Sydney, Australia, found four out of ten reported high-level anxiety symptoms, high enough to be of clinical concern. Another study, published in *The Lancet* in 2014, found half of girls and almost one third of boys have an episode of depression or anxiety in their teenage years.[121]

Whichever way you look at it, rates of depression and anxiety are rising, some due to more awareness (celebrities and even royalty are increasingly opening up about their own mental illnesses) and improved data collection, but also due to the stressors of twenty-first-century life. I doubt there would be a GP today who has never before seen a teenage girl with anxiety.

Why is there a gender gap in depression and anxiety?

For every three cases of depression, two occur in women. Anxiety shares a similar statistic.

During childhood and early puberty the rates of depression are very similar between boys and girls. From puberty onwards a gender gap appears and remains well into old age. Women and men also report different types and intensity of symptoms. Compared to men, women with depression are more likely to report loss of appetite and sleepiness, low energy, fatigue and pain.

The adult males of our species suffer from depression too, but they're slightly more likely to be diagnosed with what are called 'externalising disorders' such as drug and alcohol abuse, violence or aggression.[122] Girls and women tend to develop what are called 'internalising' disorders and often for the first time around adolescence. These include panic disorder, phobias, social anxiety disorder, obsessive-compulsive disorder and eating disorders, and post-traumatic stress disorder (PTSD). Once again, it is worth reminding you these are *average differences* and there is plenty of overlap between the sexes.

If women are more vulnerable than men to depression and anxiety, the obvious question to ask is: *Why?*

Hold on tight – the answer to this is complex because multiple interacting bottom-up, outside-in and top-down elements are responsible.

In a 2016 *Lancet Psychiatry* series on women's mental health, Christine Kuehner, a professor of clinical psychology and psychotherapy at the University of Heidelberg in Mannheim, Germany, identified the following causes for the gender gap in depression:[122]

- ♀ Genes and sex hormones.
- ♀ Women's dampened stress response.
- ♀ Women's lower self-esteem and higher tendency for body shame and rumination.
- ♀ Higher rates of experienced violence and childhood sexual abuse.
- ♀ Lack of gender equality and discrimination.

Depression – the basics

Feeling sad or lacklustre from time to time is part of being human. Sometimes symptoms are mild and caused by poor lifestyle choices, and can be treated with vigorous walking, a healthier diet and a good night's sleep. Other times depression is deep and dark, has no apparent cause, the intensity of symptoms is seriously distressing and unmanageable, and it needs professional treatment. I like to explain it by saying depression comes in many shades of blue.

If you've never suffered from depression, but would like to peer into the mind of someone who has, set aside half an hour to watch Andrew Solomon's 2013 TED talk 'Depression, the secret we share'.

Solomon, a professor of clinical psychology at Columbia University, says, 'day to day life simply became hard work. I would decide I should have lunch and then I would think, *But I'd have to get the food out and put it on a plate and cut it up and chew it and swallow it*, and it felt to me like the Stations of the Cross.' He says what often gets lost in descriptions of depression is your residual self-awareness about the undesirability of your mental state. 'Yet you are nonetheless in its grip and you are unable to figure out any way around it.'[123]

Beyondblue summarises the key symptoms of depression as:

- ♀ **Behaviours** such as not going out anymore, withdrawing from family and friends, relying on alcohol and sedatives, and not doing usual enjoyable activities.
- ♀ **Feeling** overwhelmed, irritable, lacking in confidence, indecisive, miserable or sad.
- ♀ **Thoughts** such as 'I'm a failure.' 'Nothing good ever happens to me.' 'Life's not worth living.' 'People would be better off without me.'
- ♀ **Physical symptoms** such as feeling tired all the time, sleep problems, change of appetite, weight loss or gain.[124]

Anxiety – the basics

Anxiety and depression often go hand in hand. They can occur simultaneously and reinforce one another, or one can lead to the other. Roughly half of people diagnosed with depression will meet the criteria for anxiety.

Anxiety is the most common mental health condition globally.[125] One in three women and one in five men will experience anxiety at some point in their lives.

Anxiety stems from the abnormal regulation of fear. Fear is a complex mind–body response to a perceived threat. We evolved fear to stay safe, so feelings of fear enable us to fight or flee and survive danger. When fear persists, or is out of proportion to the reality of the threat, and gets in the way of you living your life, you may have an anxiety disorder.

Beyondblue points out that the symptoms of anxiety often develop slowly over time and, given we all experience worry or anxiousness at various points in our lives, it can be hard to know how much is too much. Looking back on my biology exam panic attack, this rings true. My anxiety was stealthy and by the time I was in the throes of the panic attack it was too late to do anything about it.[126]

There are a few different types of anxiety disorder that you could be formally diagnosed with, including generalised anxiety, phobias, separation anxiety and panic disorder. Obsessive compulsive disorder and PTSD are two other conditions where anxiety is prominent.

While each anxiety condition has its own unique features, beyondblue summarises some common symptoms as:

- ♀ **Behaviours** such as avoidance of situations that make you feel anxious which can impact on study, work or social life.
- ♀ **Feelings and thoughts** such as excessive fear, worry, catastrophising, or obsessive thinking.
- ♀ **Physical symptoms** such as panic attacks, hot and cold flashes, racing heart, tightening of the chest, quick breathing, restlessness, or feeling tense, wound up and edgy.

Enduring mental wellbeing is rare

Mental health statistics get sliced, diced and interpreted in multiple ways, and rarely make for good news. So, who exactly is most at risk? Teens? LGBTI people? Middle-aged men? New mothers? Indigenous people? The elderly?

Dare I suggest all of us?

Experiencing a mental health condition at some point during the first half of your life is the norm, not the exception. People whose lives remain free from mental disorder are, in fact, remarkably rare.

This rather startling finding comes from the Dunedin Study, in which Richie Poulton and colleagues found that eighty-three per cent of people experience some form of mental illness by the age of forty. Less than one in five of us experience enduring mental wellbeing.[127]

Poulton and his colleagues write: 'readers may reasonably doubt the claim that the experience of diagnosable mental disorder is near universal.' Because their claim is so astonishing, and you may be doubtful too, it's worth spending time looking at how the finding came about.

Mental health statistics are often drawn from a particular population at a given point in time. For example, 'Danish people who received treatment in a psychiatric setting between 2000 and 2012', or 'The one in fourteen of Australians aged four to seventeen who experienced an anxiety disorder in 2015'.[128]

Furthermore, cases can only be counted if they're reported, and because plenty of people never seek treatment, their medical records are incomplete or inaccurate. Sometimes studies rely on asking people to remember if they've ever suffered from depression, and they forget. Asking people to recall events from decades earlier is a notoriously unreliable way to gather health histories. Issues with bias and reporting mean that estimates of mental illness are usually lower than actuality.

Because investigations such as the Dunedin Study meet and interview participants repeatedly over decades, there are fewer cracks for the data to fall into. Dunedin Study members have been visiting the centre every few years since they were born. At ages eleven, thirteen, fifteen, eighteen, twenty-one, twenty-six, thirty-two and thirty-eight, mental health specialists have evaluated members for symptoms of eleven common diagnoses including anxiety, depression, schizophrenia, substance abuse, attention deficit disorder and PTSD.

Of the 988 members, eighty-three per cent met the criteria for a mental health diagnosis at one or two visits up to age forty.

Only *seventeen per cent* were 'completely psychiatrically healthy' at every visit.

To be honest, I found this finding both thrilling and depressing. It finally made sense why mental health campaigns such as R U OK? Day strike a chord, or why many people find mindfulness and meditation useful. At the same time, I couldn't get my head around the idea that we should consider mental illness as 'normal'. Does this needlessly pathologise the shades of blue we all experience?

I talked over the findings with Poulton, who proposes we consider an episode of mental disorder similarly to how we'd consider a bad case of flu, kidney stones or a broken bone – all serious but recoverable conditions that are highly prevalent and may need medical attention or time to heal.

Rather than there be cause for concern around overdiagnosis and overmedicalisation of mental illness, Poulton hopes his findings reduce stigma and victim blaming. 'People who are mentally ill really get crapped on by society,' he said candidly. 'We can talk as much as we like about mental health and mental illness in the media, but the stigma remains for many people, who then fail to ask for help.'

As expected, the healthy seventeen per cent came from childhood backgrounds virtually free of the well-known predictors of poor mental health such as childhood abuse, poverty or illness. These childhood predictors were common in the group who experienced more severe cases of schizophrenia, mania or PTSD.

A key comparison in the study was between the healthy seventeen per cent and those who experienced mild bouts of anxiety or depression – they were no more or less likely to come from early childhood adversity or trauma. The difference between the two groups was childhood temperament, and a relative absence of family psychiatric history. The seventeen per cent scored low on Poulton's marker, 'negative emotional reactivity'. As children they had few emotional difficulties, lots of friends and showed superior levels of willpower or self-control. 'You'd never describe these kids as loners, frequent worriers, sad or tearful,' he said.

You might wonder, does *enduring* mental health matter? Have the seventeen per cent won a wellbeing lottery?

As you might expect, the seventeen per cent went on to achieve more 'desirable' life outcomes – they stayed in education longer, landed better-paying jobs, and had higher-quality relationships (they rated respect and fairness, emotional intimacy and trust, and open communication in their relationships as high). They'd be the type of people the psychology literature would describe as 'flourishing'. This study draws a nice parallel to other reports of rare physical health, such as centenarians who manage to live to 100 years or older with unusually enduring *physical* health.

Clearly there is a strong advantage gained in life by those who escape even transient mild issues with depression and anxiety. Such advantage starts in childhood and snowballs with age. The role of abundant social support in childhood to buffer against adversity cannot be underestimated. Poulton points out that human bonds formed at any stage of life can be transformative, and there is always the potential for warm, benevolent relationships later in life to repair the damage done in childhood.

What does a depressed brain look like?

There's no blood test or biological markers for depression or anxiety. A psychiatrist friend of mine explained to me that she diagnoses depression based on what people tell her about their feelings, how they're behaving and what they're thinking.

Could a brain scan diagnose depression, or predict who might become depressed in the future?

Data compiled from brain scans of many thousands of people with depression collected by the international consortium ENIGMA identified a few key abnormalities in the structure and operation of depressed brains.[129] ENIGMA was set up to promote collaboration between disparate research groups all working on the same problem. Their simple aim is to obtain the large sample sizes necessary to detect what are often tiny differences between healthy and unhealthy brains.

The depression research arm of ENIGMA is led by Lianne Schmaal, who tells me this is the largest coordinated worldwide meta-analysis of brain structure changes in people with depression. 'Now we have robust and reliable evidence for the small and subtle differences that exist,' she says.

So far Schmaal's team has crunched the numbers for the effects of depression on subcortical structures and cortical grey matter; the white matter data is still being processed. A comparison of 1728 people with depression and 7199 healthy controls found adults with recurrent depression had an ever so slightly shrunken hippocampus. The hippocampus is an area of the brain responsible for emotion processing and forming new memories. Hippocampal 'shrinkage' (a term Schmaal doesn't like using) was most pronounced among those people whose depression started in their teenage years.

People with depression also had an ever-so-slightly smaller amygdala, although the difference wasn't as noticeable as hippocampal shrinkage. Involvement of the amygdala in depression should come as no surprise – it is intimately involved in processing emotions, especially fear.

Schmaal's second study examined the cortical grey matter of 2148 depressed people and 7957 healthy controls from twenty sites around the world. Adults with depression had an ever-so-slightly thinner cortex (specifically in orbitofrontal cortex, cingulate, insula and temporal lobes) compared to healthy controls. A key feature of these regions is their close interaction with the amygdala and hippocampus.

Do depressed people have brain structures that tend to be 'shrunken' or thinner to begin with, or does depression cause the damage? Some ENIGMA researchers propose that it's likely depression causes the shrinkage, as shrinkage was only present in people with long-lasting or severe depression, not those with a one-off episode or milder cases.

Do depressed brains work differently from healthy brains?

People with depression tend to have detectable differences in the electrical activity in certain parts of their brain. In particular, levels of neural activity in the PFC and amygdala sometimes differ between healthy and depressed people.

In healthy adults, top-down PFC modulation of the amygdala keeps emotions in check. Brain imaging studies show that with depression the PFC is *less active* and the amygdala are *over active* compared to normal. People with depression have what can be thought of as a 'trigger-happy' amygdala.[130]

A trigger-happy amygdala that overreacts to negative emotional stimuli fits with the theory (just one of many) that depressed people look at their world with a strong negative emotional bias. Rather than the rose-tinted glasses through which an optimist would view the world, someone with depression sees the world in shades of grey.

The dysfunctional dialogue between the limbic system and PFC is seen in both depressed adult women and in teenage girls. One reason that teens have a tendency to get depressed is because the lines of communication between the PFC and limbic system are still developing.

To be clear, we're not able to diagnose depression by scanning someone's brain (especially if they've not been depressed for long). Differences detected by ENIGMA were so subtle they could only be spotted when many thousands of scans were combined. Just as we cannot tell if you're a man or a woman by your MRI, we cannot tell if you're depressed or not either.

Lianne Schmaal tells me that her research shows what neuroscience calls 'neural correlates' of depression and that 'it is not a diagnostic tool'. She hopes her data will eventually be able to predict if someone with depression or anxiety would respond to a particular antidepressant, or to a talking therapy.

Is depression caused by a chemical imbalance in the brain?

Let's zoom in and look at depressed and anxious brains under a microscope.

In his TED talk Andrew Solomon describes his experiences with antidepressants. People ask him if his 'happy pills' make him feel happy. They don't make him 'feel happy' he says. 'But I don't feel sad about having to eat lunch, and I don't feel sad about my answering machine, and I don't feel sad about taking a shower.'[123]

Antidepressant drugs are one of the most widely used treatments for depression. There is considerable evidence they work well for some adults with severe depression. For other adults, particularly those with mild to moderate depression, they tend to work no better than a placebo. In this instance, psychological treatments and lifestyle changes such as regular vigorous exercise may be just as effective.[131]

Modern antidepressants are thought to work on a trio of brain chemicals called the monoamines: serotonin, noradrenaline and dopamine. Serotonin is involved in mood and emotion, noradrenaline is involved in stress and attention, and dopamine tells us what we want and is involved in motivation and reward.

The idea that monoamines might have something to do with depression emerged back in the 1950s. Doctors noticed that reserpine, a chemical derived from the rauwolfia plant, widely used in India to treat high blood pressure, *caused* depression. Reserpine blocks the initial packaging up of monoamines into vesicles for release at synapses. It was reasoned that depression must be due to too little monoamine being packaged for release. Support for this idea came from another discovery that drugs that slow breakdown of released monoamines in the synapse cured depression in some people.

A seemingly logical hypothesis thus emerged: depression is due to a deficiency of one or more monoamines. If you increase monoamine levels (with drugs), you'll cure depression.

SSRIs are one type of antidepressant that block the action of the molecule serotonin transport protein (SERT) in the synapse. Neurons run rather economical electrochemical enterprises: once they release their chemical packages of serotonin into the synapse, SERT acts like a mini vacuum cleaner, immediately sucking serotonin back up into the neuron from which it was released. This simultaneously terminates serotonin's effect and enables it to be repackaged and re-used. SSRIs act rather like a large wad of paper clogging up the SERT vacuum cleaner hose, preventing the reuptake of serotonin. The longer serotonin lingers in the synapse, the stronger its effect.

It is important to note that while SSRIs make all the difference in the world for many people, they don't work for everyone. This is one of many puzzles and weaknesses in the 'depression as a biochemical imbalance' hypothesis.

Another puzzle is the time lag between treatment and symptom improvement. Antidepressants act in the brain to increase monoamine levels pretty much the day you pop the first pill. But changes in mood (if they occur at all) take two or three weeks to kick in.

Bearing in mind we can't yet measure neurotransmitter levels in the brains of living humans (all our data comes from lab animals), we're in the dark about how much monoamine levels need to change to alter mood. Curiously, a drug called tianeptine that enhances the action of SERT, thereby lowering serotonin levels, has been used as a treatment for depression.

Another criticism of the chemical imbalance hypothesis is that it treats depression as a purely brain chemical problem, and fails to recognise there are biological, psychological, social and spiritual causes. But I've never been convinced this criticism is valid – research into genes, inflammation, social isolation and stress as causes of depression is well established. Neuroscience is far more broad ranging than critics assume!

Of interest to readers will be that serotonin acts somewhat differently in women and men. Women manufacture less serotonin than men and have fewer serotonin receptors. And some (but not all) studies have found that SSRIs are more effective among women than among men.[132] Sex differences in serotonin emerge at puberty and disappear among the elderly, suggesting a role for reproductive hormones.

Experiments in male and female rodents have shown ovarian hormones alter levels of electrical activity in serotonergic neurons. Oestrogen and progesterone alter serotonin synthesis, breakdown and removal from the synapse.

Clearly, treating depression has proven way more difficult than simply increasing serotonin levels by blocking neurotransmitter reuptake. Altered levels of monoamines may not necessarily be the *cause* any more than a smaller than normal hippocampus is the *cause* of depression. Rather, biochemical signatures may be another 'neural correlate' of depression.

Is there a gene for depression?

Twins share parents, the womb and a childhood home, and identical twins share 100 per cent of their DNA. Studies of identical and fraternal twins are often used to assess how much genes versus environment matters, and such studies have shown the genetic risk of developing clinical depression is about forty per cent. That leaves another sixty per cent due to other outside-in or top-down causes.

Gene-environment (GxE) studies investigate whether our genes moderate our susceptibility to experiences such as stressful life events.

Poulton likes to explain GxE interactions using his finding that cannabis hikes schizophrenia risk in certain people. People with a particular variation of the gene 'COMT' (G) who used cannabis during adolescence (E) are eleven times more likely to go on to develop schizophrenia than people without the gene. The COMT gene, which is found in only twenty-five per cent of the population, confers vulnerability to developing psychosis but *only* if you use cannabis during your adolescent years. The seventy-five per cent of people without the gene don't experience the same dramatically increased risk, nor do those *with* the gene who smoke cannabis in adulthood. ('If you want to smoke weed, wait till you're an adult,' is his sage advice.)[133]

GxE interactions have been used to explain the genetic differences between dandelion and orchid children. Recall in chapter 2 I introduced the idea that some children are more resilient and others more vulnerable to stress. Unlike their robust resilient dandelion peers, orchid children and the highly sensitive adults they grow into are less resilient. Orchids have the potential for either weakness or flourishing depending on how they're nurtured.[134]

Just as the COMT gene confers vulnerability to psychosis under very specific circumstances, a variation of an 'orchid gene' is thought to increase susceptibility to depression in response to extreme stress. Surprisingly, the orchid gene is the very same gene that codes for SERT – the serotonin mini vacuum cleaner blocked by SSRIs.

We inherit different lengths of the SERT gene from our parents. You might inherit two longs, two shorts, or a long and a short copy. SERT is dose dependent – having one or two copies of short SERT doesn't guarantee depression, but *if* you're exposed to stress or trauma you're far more likely to get depressed than the resilient people who inherited two long copies.

SERT is now one of the most well-studied genes in mental health. Short SERT copies are implicated in everything from depression to neuroticism, to having a 'trigger-happy' amygdala, to blushing and social anxiety.

The Dunedin Study found that people with short SERT copies were more likely to be depressed and even become suicidal if, *and only if* – they were exposed to a stressful event or childhood maltreatment. People with short SERT who were not exposed to severe stress displayed exceptional resilience.[135]

Of course, science is never so neat and tidy – the case of SERT and genetic sensitivity to stress has proven controversial. A meta-analysis published while I was writing this chapter failed to replicate the early studies implicating short SERT as the go-between for stress and depression. The study included a whopping 43 165 subjects and was a collaborative effort between multiple groups that, like ENIGMA, are dedicated to sharing existing data to improve the reliability of research findings.[136]

Incidentally, the mega meta-analysis did find strong evidence for two risk factors for developing depression: being female and life stress. Looks like we're back to where we started.

Is the depression gender gap due to sex hormones?

Clearly being a woman increases risk of depression. Who is going to argue with a meta-analysis of 43 165 subjects? Does this mean we're back to blaming our hormones?

Oestrogen may improve mood

It often comes as a surprise to learn that oestrogen promotes brain health and improves mood. Clinical studies indicate that our mental health is most fragile when oestrogen levels are dwindling, both over the course of the month and the course of the lifespan.

For example, women have a lower incidence of schizophrenia compared to men before the age of forty-five. After age forty-five, twice as many women as men are diagnosed. High levels of oestrogen in young fertile women are thought to delay the onset of the disease.[137]

Such episodes are rare, but sudden withdrawal of oestrogen can cause psychosis in women who have just given birth, which is when oestogen levels drop 1000-fold. And psychotic episodes are reported in women being treated with the breast cancer drug tamoxifen, which blocks the action of oestrogen.[137]

Less dramatically, we've seen that blunting our natural oestrogen levels with the contraceptive pill dampens vitality, wellbeing and positive mood, and low levels of oestrogen are also blamed for the symptoms of PMDD.

Rodent studies have found that oestrogen promotes neuronal sprouting, enhances synaptic plasticity and increases axon myelination. Oestrogen acts as an anti-inflammatory, an antioxidant, slows neuronal cell death, and improves cerebral blood flow and glucose metabolism. Furthermore, oestrogen modulates the activity of the brain's own chemical fertiliser, brain-derived neurotrophic factor.

If our mental health is so clearly vulnerable to *withdrawal* of oestrogen, does this mean there is a place for oestrogen replacement as a therapy?

Jayashri Kulkarni believes so. Kulkarni has conducted trials and found that women with schizophrenia being treated with antipsychotics who receive additional doses of oestrogen via a skin patch improve faster than women who only take antipsychotics. Kulkarni is so convinced about the positive effects of oestrogen that instead of blaming 'hormones' on mood, she likes to say, 'Isn't she doing well because of her hormones. Maybe we should give them to him!'[138]

Progesterone may exacerbate anxiety and PTSD

Of course, in healthy, naturally cycling women, oestrogen doesn't work alone. Rising levels of oestrogen precede and then overlap with rising levels of progesterone and it can be difficult to draw conclusions about the exact role of each hormone (one good reason why studies of the menstrual cycle and the pill are so hard to decipher).

To help unpack the role of ovarian hormones in depression and anxiety, I met up with clinical psychologist and University of New South Wales (UNSW) neuroscientist Bronwyn Graham. Graham runs a program where she combines traditional laboratory research in rodents with clinical work in humans.

Graham told me she started her research career as a 'typical neuroscientist', only studying male rats because females with their fluctuating hormones added too much 'noise' to the data. She also admitted to thinking sex difference research was 'lazy science'. Curiosity eventually got the better of her and she realised that rather than dismissing the variance female rats introduced to data, it might be more interesting to shift her focus to studying the 'noise' itself.

Lucky for us, because Graham's research has shown hormonal fluctuations influence women's susceptibility to anxiety in response to stress and vulnerability to PTSD.[139]

PTSD is a particular set of reactions that can develop in people who have been through a traumatic event which threatens their life or safety or that of others around them. This could be a car or other serious accident, assault, or disasters such as a bushfire or flood. As a result, the people experience feelings of intense fear, helplessness or horror.[126] Compared to males, girls and women are twice as likely to develop PTSD after experiencing a traumatic incident.

As I drove to meet Graham in late May 2017, news filtered through on my car radio of a terrorist attack on a pop concert in Manchester, England. Over coffee our discussion inevitably turned to the trauma trajectory the girls and young women at the concert would then be facing.

Graham explained to me that after an horrific event like a terrorist attack, the vast majority of people experience some post-traumatic symptoms. For example, girls who were at the concert in Manchester would be doing their best to avoid thinking about the event, but at the same time they'd be having unwanted and recurring memories, often in the form of vivid images and nightmares. They'd be having intense emotional or physical reactions, such as sweating, heart palpitations or panic; they'd be jumpy and hyper alert, would have trouble sleeping and feel emotionally numb. Over time, about eighty to ninety per cent spontaneously recover. Who develops full-blown PTSD depends on life history, previous mental health problems, genetic vulnerability and the availability of social support.

Intriguingly, menstrual cycle phase at the time of trauma may facilitate the development of PTSD. It's becoming increasingly apparent that sex hormones interact with stress hormones to affect our response to trauma.[140]

Graham hypothesises that trauma coinciding with premenstrual low oestrogen and high progesterone contributes to a more deeply encoded memory of the event. Memory over-consolidation, as it is called, is thought to generate unwanted or distressing intrusive memories of trauma. Recall in chapter 4 that we looked at research showing emotional memories tended to be more durable during the low-oestrogen and high-progesterone luteal phase of the menstrual cycle.

Oestrogen, as we know, is protective and around ovulation it reduces anxiety. In girls and women with high (versus low) oestrogen at the time of the trauma, fear extinction is more likely. Fear extinction is when the scary memories gradually become less upsetting and intrusive over time. Two other studies support Graham's intriguing hypothesis.

In one study, 138 women who were admitted to Westmead Hospital in Sydney, Australia, following a traumatic accident (most admissions were from car accidents, but also falls and non-sexual assaults) were assessed for PTSD symptoms, including flashbacks. Hormone levels were inferred by asking women when they got their last period. Women were more likely to experience flashback memories if they were in the high-progesterone luteal phase of their cycle at the time of trauma. One in five (twenty-two per cent) of women in the luteal phase experienced flashback memories compared to less than one in ten (nine per cent) who were in another phase of their cycle.[141]

A second study published in the *Journal of Forensic Nursing* followed up 111 sexual-assault survivors six months after their trauma. The researchers found that those who had taken an emergency contraceptive (also known as the morning after pill) or who were already taking the pill showed fewer symptoms of PTSD.[142] Similar findings from other groups have also shown the pill blunts women's responses to psychosocial stress.[143] As Graham explains, both forms of contraception suppress women's natural levels of progesterone, thereby diminishing memory overconsolidation and intrusive memories.

As fascinating as these findings on hormones and PTSD are, like much work on the interaction between the pill and the brain, research is pre-pubertal. It's difficult to translate the findings on menstrual cycle phase, oral contraceptive use and development of PTSD or anxiety into real-world advice. For example, we simply cannot recommend the pill as a 'vaccine' against PTSD.

Bronwyn Graham is well aware of this and told me that when she puts on her clinical psychologist hat she doesn't focus on the myriad reasons *why* she has a patient under her care. Rather, she focuses on helping that person get better. 'I often say to people that if you go to hospital with a broken leg, the doctors don't spend hours trying to figure out how and why you fell out of a tree. They spend time looking at the break and how it can be fixed,' she said. 'It's the same with mental health.'

The inner mean girl

Few of us would consider speaking to our friends, children or even pets in the same way we speak to ourselves. Negative self-talk contributes to the gender gap in depression – the voice is louder and meaner in girls and women than in boys and men.

I found one line of research on early puberty and depression particularly interesting, because it looked at the propensity for girls to ruminate – that is, to 'overthink' or mentally chew over intense emotional experiences, and their possible causes and consequences, rather than coming up with proactive solutions. Rumination is a well-known risk factor for depression and leads to hopelessness, pessimism and self-criticism. Gender differences in the tendency to guilt and shame oneself emerge, as you might expect, during adolescence, when they are especially focused on body dissatisfaction.

There is a saying that worrying is like a rocking chair: it will give you something to do, but it won't get you anywhere. Teenage girls, especially, get caught in a trap when they find a close friend to co-ruminate with. Such friendships have the benefits of promoting emotional closeness, but discussing, rehashing and speculating about problems together can stress girls out even more thereby exacerbating depression.

Another top-down mediator of depression is personality. Psychologists measure what they call the Big Five personality traits: openness, conscientiousness, extroversion, agreeableness and neuroticism. Each trait is a continuum and describes your tendencies, habits of thought and ways of relating to others and the world. Someone who scores high on negative emotionality or neuroticism would typically be anxious, highly strung, tense, nervy and prone to stewing over things, versus someone who is emotionally stable and doesn't react to stress. Compare the cool, calm, detached indifference of James Bond versus the anxious and nervy George Costanza character.[122]

The Dunedin Study has found that young adults who score low on traits of conscientiousness and agreeableness, and high on neuroticism, are more prone to developing depression.

Depression is a stress-related disorder

You may have noticed that in each of the preceding sections the unifying theme (besides being female) is stress. It could be said that nature (in the form of genes or hormones or personality or social support or biological sex) loads the bullet and stress fires the gun.

How does a stressful event get under our skin?

We all respond to stress in a variety of ways, and whether an event is a 'stressor' varies from person to person. What I may perceive as relatively benign might be construed as very threatening to you and elicit a biological stress response and vice versa. I remember visiting my family in Christchurch in the days following the massive September 2010 earthquake, which occurred in the middle of the night. I was sitting on the couch with my sister one evening as she described feeling deeply unsettled and frightened as it grew dark. Despite knowing earthquakes were no more likely to occur at night than in the day, in her hypervigilant state, darkness was a new stressor.

We feel stressed when real or imagined pressures exceed our perceived ability to cope. A major factor in dealing with stress is having access to practical, social or emotional resources to prop you up. Sometimes it's not so much the actual event itself but how it makes us feel and for how long we feel helpless afterwards. Problems arise when we're repeatedly stressed or stressed for prolonged periods.

How exactly does a stressor act to elicit a biological response that leads to depression? To understand, we'll need to take a closer look at how our stress response works and how it integrates body and brain.

The neurobiology of stress

There are two biological pathways that work together to mediate the stress response: the sympathetic nervous system (SNS) and the HPA axis. These two systems exist in our bodies to maintain physiological balance or, as scientists say, homeostasis.

The SNS is the front-line 'fight or flight' responder and activates the adrenal medulla of the adrenal glands, which sit like little berets on top of the kidneys. The adrenal medulla release adrenaline and noradrenaline into the bloodstream, fuelling our ability to 'fight' or 'flee'.

The HPA axis is slower to respond but is longer lasting.

The HPA axis consists of the hypothalamus, the pituitary and the adrenal cortex, which is where cortisol – perhaps one of our most maligned and misunderstood of hormones – is made.

Cortisol has an undeserved bad reputation. I find it useful to think of cortisol as the Goldilocks hormone. You need just the right amount – too little or too much and you have health problems. Like all hormones, cortisol is merely a key to unlock a door. The lock is the glucocorticoid receptor. How cortisol acts depends on glucocorticoid receptors, especially their numbers and where they're located. The receptors mediate HPA-axis negative feedback, that is, the ability of cortisol to inhibit its own secretion.

In some people with depression, malfunctioning glucocorticoid receptors cause the HPA-axis to become *over*-active resulting in excessive cortisol flooding the body and brain. This is called 'glucocorticoid resistance'.

In other groups of depressed people the HPA-axis is *under-active*. Women make up a large proportion of this group. Compared to men, our stress response is slightly blunted. As you might expect, the HPA and HPO axes are interconnected. We know that a stress-induced activation of the HPA-axis slows oestrogen production and, in turn, oestrogen can enhance HPA-axis responses.[140]

Sex differences in the stress response emerge at puberty. One explanation for the rise in depression rates in teenage girls is the maturation of the interconnected female HPA and HPO axes.

Dutch researcher Albertine Oldehinkel has perfected a rather 'nasty' social stress experiment called the Groningen Social Stress Test that shows how males and females react differently to stress.[144] Once volunteers arrive in the lab, have their blood pressure monitored and a saliva sample tested for cortisol, Oldehinkel abruptly asks them to present an off-the-cuff six-minute public speech about their lives. She tells them it will be recorded to be evaluated and rated by their friends. Immediately after the speech she then asks the volunteer to stand in front of a group of people and subtract the number seventeen repeatedly, starting with 1327, and all the while she shouts instructions such as 'Stop wiggling your hands' or 'You are too slow, be as quick as you can, we are running out of time!' As you'd expect, blood pressure and salivary cortisol levels shoot up immediately after the test!

Oldehinkel's work has shown teenage boys and men tend to display larger cortisol responses to social stress than teenage girls and women. These sex differences emerge at puberty, disappear at menopause, and for women vary during the menstrual cycle and if they're on the pill. 'We propose that particularly blunted cortisol responses to stress are associated with a high likelihood of depression after stressful life events occurrence,' writes Oldehinkel. Multiple studies have demonstrated the counterintuitive result that high cortisol levels during stress are associated with lower risk of subsequent depression.

Oldehinkel suggests that cortisol prepares the body to face stressful situations by, among other things, increasing glucose levels; for some reason this is up-regulated in men. 'Women's blunted cortisol reaction to stress may therefore result in decreased energy supply and fatigue, which in turn could induce other depressive symptoms,' she says. 'An alternative explanation could be that blunted stress responses signal dysfunctional coping strategies, which can lead to feelings of discomfort and lack of control following the stressful experience.'

Is depression due to inflammation?

'Inflammation' is the health buzzword of the moment. There is growing evidence that inflammation – already implicated in heart disease, obesity, and metabolic disorders – is involved in brain diseases, including Alzheimer's disease, multiple sclerosis and perhaps depression.

The brain has its own resident immune system consisting of microglia that migrate into the brain during embryonic development. As well as resident microglia, an intimate *tête-à-tête* exists between the brain and peripheral immune system.

Some researchers hypothesise that not only physical threats like viruses or injury but also social challenges, stress and adversity trigger the production of 'pro-inflammatory cytokines' – messenger molecules that orchestrate the immune response to injury and infection.

Cytokine levels are altered in anxiety and depression. Evidence from both human and animal studies has found that injecting inflammatory cytokines causes depressive symptoms.[145] One clinical trial found that depressed people who had not responded to antidepressants improved after being treated with an anti-inflammatory drug, but only if they already had increased inflammatory cytokine levels.[146]

From an evolutionary perspective, successful defence against pathogens involved not only the activation of our immune system but also behaviours such as hypervigilance against future attack or hiding away (in bed with a pillow over your head) if sick or wounded. It's proposed 'sickness' behaviours which closely mimic depression were beneficial for the survival of women, because we were mostly involved in homely activities such as child care, whereas men were the adventurous hunters and providers of food and protection.

So, is depression a side effect of inflammation?

Maybe. While there may be a connection between inflammation and depression, we can't say for sure that one leads directly to the other. Not everyone who suffers from depression has evidence of inflammation. Likewise, not all people with high levels of inflammation develop depression. As we've seen, depression depends on a complex interplay of a spectrum of risks and resilience which are present to varying degrees and in different combinations in everyone.

'One thing is for sure,' writes Carmine Pariante, a researcher with an interest in stress, inflammation and depression. 'Depression and mental health problems in general can no longer be seen only as disorders of the mind, or indeed only as disorders of the brain. The strong impact of the immune system on emotions and behaviour demonstrates that mental health is the health of the whole body.'[147]

Stress and gender issues

Globally, girls and women are at greater risk from gender-based violence including rape, forced marriage, intimate partner violence, genital mutilation and childhood sexual abuse than males. Childhood sexual abuse estimates indicate a prevalence of about one in five girls and just under one in ten boys. These estimates are thought to be conservative and the WHO reports put the figure closer to seventy per cent in some countries.[148]

'Part of the gender gap might be explained by heightened exposure to severe adversity, particularly childhood sexual abuse and other violence against women and girls,' writes Kuehner in *Lancet Psychiatry*.[122]

Kuehner points out that gender inequality in terms of political participation, economic autonomy and reproductive rights affects the gender ratio in depression. For example, one study found women living in US states with lower gender equality reported more depressive symptoms than women living in states with higher gender equality.[149] Similar findings have been reported in Europe.[150]

The global Women's March of 2017 and mottos that have sprung rapidly into our collective consciousness ('Nevertheless, she persisted' being my personal favourite) highlight how far we have to go to achieve gender equality and recognition of girls' and women's rights. The social media #MeToo campaign that swept the globe in late 2017, during which women who had been sexually harassed or assaulted wrote 'Me too' as a status update, suggests the WHO estimates are likely accurate.

You're depressed or anxious – now what?

At this point it's worth considering whether neuroscience can shed any light on mental illness at all. There has always been criticism in psychology and psychiatry about the 'seduction of reductionism', and whether we can explain or cure mental illness by looking at its neural or genetic underpinnings. From my perspective, considering mental illness through a neuroscience lens isn't an attempt to offer answers but just one of many lenses through which to view the problem.

Not all treatments work for all people all of the time

There are many different approaches to treat depression and anxiety. They can be loosely divided up into:

Medical treatments
- ♀ Antidepressants and/or anti-anxiolytics.
- ♀ Electrical stimulation, e.g. electroconvulsive therapy, or transcranial magnetic stimulation.

Psychological therapies
- ♀ Talking therapies, e.g. cognitive behavioural therapy.
- ♀ Mindfulness-based therapies.
- ♀ Relationship therapy.

Lifestyle therapies
- ♀ Exercise, dietary changes, massage, sleep deprivation, mindfulness and meditation and so on.

Any reputable doctor or therapist will tell you that just because a treatment is shown to work scientifically, that does not mean it will work equally well for everyone. In other words: not all treatments work for all people all of the time.

The world of wellbeing is full of claims and counterclaims, accusations and conflicting information about mind and brain health. I suggest that if someone claims they have *the* one-size-fits-all solution to your mental health problem, that you're 'weak' or 'not a feminist' or 'opting out of your healing journey by trying antidepressants' or any other such stigmatising or non-supportive comment, then run the other way. I also find the use of the word 'truth' to be a red flag. Find someone who'll help find the right solution for you.

Beyondblue clearly states, 'While [a treatment] might work for the average person, some people will have complications, side-effects or incompatibilities with their lifestyle. The best strategy is to try an approach that works for most people and that you are comfortable with. If you do not recover quickly enough, or experience problems with the treatment, then try another.'

Another factor to consider is your belief system. Treatments are more likely to work if you believe they will, which is why placebo effects are powerful. Curiously, the most powerful ingredient of the placebo effect is the therapeutic relationship. Once again human connection, love and affection are the ultimate buffers for stress and the solution to many of our ills.

7.

Sex, Love and Neurobiology

IF YOU MIX A GIN AND TONIC IN A ROOM LIT BY ULTRAVIOLET LIGHT, your drink will glow a brilliant blue. This is because tonic contains a chemical called quinine, originally used to treat malaria, and when exposed to the right wavelength of light the chemical fluoresces. After being told this fact by a university lecturer, my best friend and I spent much of the late 1990s promenading around clubs and parties with glasses of glowing blue gin in our hands. They acted as our conversation starters, our lures, our tools of woo.

In January 1999, my G&T and I were prowling round a house on Banbury Road in Oxford when we caught the eye of a young Irish economist with a smile as brilliant as my gin. 'What are you drinking?' he asked. 'Let me tell you about ultraviolet spectrum of light,' I replied. The attraction was instant. We went on to discuss interest rates (I never understood the difference between interest paid and earned, and he patiently explained) and synapses. During our gin-soaked conversation he learned 'synapse' is Latin for 'clasp, join together, tie or bind, to be in connection with'. Prescient words, because we've been bound together ever since. Yes, I seduced my husband with the language of science – first with physics, then with neurobiology.

Love has inspired great works of art and literature, and countless song lyrics, and forms the foundations of our families, so I understand it seems almost sacrilegious to consider it through the lens of neuroscience. Yet love is profoundly biological and deeply affects our bodies and minds. In the absence of loving relationships, babies fail to flourish. Children raised in abusive homes carry psychological scars for life. Teenagers become suicidal in the face of bullying or unrequited love. New mothers lacking the so-called village of social support slip into postnatal depression. Marital status is correlated to health – on average you're better off health-wise married than single. Loneliness in the elderly has the same impact on dementia risk as smoking a pack of cigarettes a day.

Considering sex through the lens of biology is perhaps a concept we're more comfortable with. It's common to hear it's not our genitals but, rather, our brains that are our most sexual organs. Sex is perhaps the ultimate bottom-up outside-in top-down biological experience.

In this chapter, we'll explore the neurobiology of attraction, desire, the sexual response cycle and orgasms. Then we'll close the bedroom door to focus on romantic love, attachment and how social connections buffer stress.

Adolescence is a sensitive period for learning about sex

As a teen, I had a clear image in mind of my ideal guy and spent many hours dreaming about where we'd meet (often in a library, which is kind of embarrassing to admit but that was my native habitat), what beaches we'd walk along hand in hand,

and the heart-to-heart conversations we'd have. Helen Fisher, a biological anthropologist who works at the world-renowned Kinsey Institute for sex research calls this idealistic image a 'love map'. 'Long before your true love walks up to you in a classroom, at a shopping mall, in the office, at a coffee shop, or at a party or event,' says Fisher, 'you have constructed the basic elements of your ideal sweetheart.'

We start to piece together our love maps during adolescence around the same time our sexual feelings first develop. Teenage brains are very plastic, and adolescence is thus a sensitive period for learning how to navigate romantic and sexual relationships. Research has largely ignored this phase of development, and only recently have we realised that adolescence is when young women begin to explore their sexual identity, construct their love maps, and hopefully gain positive and affirming experiences that will inform both.[151]

The alchemy of attraction

What happens in our brains when we're sexually attracted to one person and not another? Why him? Why her? Why a smiling Irish economist in January 1999? Fate? Hormones? Pheromones? Complementary love maps? Or, in my case, too much gin?

One robust finding in the 'mate choice' literature is that we tend to pair up with people who are 'like us' – a phenomenon known as 'positive assortative mating'. On average (not always), we're attracted to someone of a similar age, ethnicity and socioeconomic background, someone with the same level of intelligence and education, someone who shares our values and goals, and someone physically similar. Those couples in decades-long relationships didn't morph over time to look alike; research shows they actively sought out a look-alike mate from the start. 'We're more like our partners than would be expected by chance,' University of Queensland researcher Brendan Zietsch told me.

Because I walked into an Oxford graduate party one night in January 1999, there was a high chance I'd find someone who'd match my 'love map'. And it's likely we 'positively assorted' ourselves too. When I first showed a photo of my new beau to my blue-gin partner in crime her immediate response was, 'He's *definitely* a you boy!'

As primitive as it seems, how we smell may also be part of the sexual chemistry equation. Pheromones are chemical signals that have evolved for communication with other members of the same species, and the pheromones in our sweat provide a potent clue to the owner's genes. In particular, genes code for a group of immune molecules called major histocompatibility complexes (MHCs). Here's where evolution gets devious: it turns out we're more attracted to the smell of MHCs that are most *dissimilar* to our own. Quite the opposite from what positive assortative look-alike theory would have you guess.

The Swiss 'sweaty T-shirt study' published in 1995 found that the more different a man's MHC genes are from a woman's, the more attractive he seems to her. In the study, male and female students from the University of Bern were first typed for their MHCs, then each man was given a T-shirt to wear for a couple of days and nights (they were encouraged not to shower or use deodorant). After they returned the sweaty T-shirts, the women were given six shirts to sniff and rate by preference. Ultimately, women preferred the sweaty smell of men whose MHC was most dissimilar to their own. They often remarked that they preferred shirts that reminded them of their boyfriends, both past and present, whereas unfavourable-smelling shirts tended to remind women of their fathers.[152]

Interestingly, women on the contraceptive pill showed a stronger preference for sweaty T-shirts worn by men who were most MHC-*similar*. We have a heightened sense of smell around ovulation, and it's thought this is how evolution ensures that genetic diversity is maintained. MHC-dissimilar couples are more fertile and less likely to be related. Somehow the pill interferes with this mechanism.[153]

How hormones influence mate choice and sex drive

The female sex drive waxes and wanes across the monthly cycle, peaking around ovulation. Evidence shows that fluctuation in ovarian hormones influences who we find attractive, who finds us attractive, and how frisky we feel.

Here's some research that always causes quite a stir.

A 2012 paper entertainingly titled 'Ovulation leads women to perceive sexy cads as good dads' suggests that when we're most fertile we're more likely to be attracted to the high-testosterone masculine man of 'superior genetic quality' versus the bookish nice guy who'd make a 'good husband and father'. (Note, the research is about who we're *attracted to*, not necessarily sleeping with.) In contrast, when we're on the pill, or in the luteal or bleeding phases of our cycles, we quite happily settle for the nice guy.[154]

There is data both supporting and refuting this so-called 'ovulation shift cad or dad' hypothesis. Rob Brooks, a professor of evolutionary ecology at the University of New South Wales has tracked the literature and points out that the shifts in preferences are actually pretty small. 'It's not as though you're going to be truly, madly, deeply in love with your husband the one day and furtively shagging the pool guy the next,' he says. Brooks also notes that what's more intriguing is we're still happy to jump into the sack when the chances of conceiving are nil.[155]

Feeling frisky on oestrogen

If you remember, in chapter 6 I met with researcher Bronwyn Graham, who explained that around ovulation oestrogen lowers anxiety. Female animals in oestrus hop, preen, wriggle their ears, dance, sing, change colour or display lordosis – the 'come hither' response female rodents adopt to enable males to mount – to attract a mate. Oestrogen leads to females feeling less risk averse and more willing to act in a way that encourages sexual interaction. Of course, we human women don't exactly go into heat, strip off our knickers and run around shagging every willing male in the vicinity when we ovulate, but there is good evidence to suggest that oestrogen makes us feel frisky and behave in subtle ways that display this desire to a potential mate.

In 2013 a paper published in the journal *Hormones and Behavior* described the relationship between three hormones (oestradiol, progesterone and testosterone) and women's sexual desire.[156] By now it shouldn't surprise you that this was one of the first comprehensive studies to explore desire, hormones and the menstrual cycle.

Each morning of the study, forty-three naturally cycling women (i.e. women not using hormonal contraceptives) collected a salivary sample that was used to assay their individual levels of oestradiol, progesterone and testosterone. Then the women were prompted by an app to respond to the following questions: 'Did you engage in sexual activity (intercourse or other forms of genital stimulation) with another person yesterday?' 'Who initiated the sexual activity? (You, Other person, Both)' 'Did you engage in self-stimulation (masturbation) yesterday?'

The wording of questions was important. Historically, good old-fashioned penis-in-vagina intercourse was taken as the principal indicator of women's desire. We now understand that a far more accurate measure of desire is to ask women whether or not they *felt* like having sex, if they masturbated or if they initiated sex with a partner.

When the data were crunched, the following relationships between hormones and desire were found:

- ♀ Oestradiol increased desire.
- ♀ Progesterone decreased desire.
- ♀ Testosterone had no impact on desire whatsoever.

Australian women's health researcher Professor Lorraine Dennerstein has also found a link between oestrogen and desire. For eight years she tracked a cohort of 226 women as they transitioned from early to late menopause. As we'll learn in chapter 9, levels of ovarian hormones decline during menopause. Each woman's hormone levels and sexual desire were charted and Dennerstein found that oestrogen was indeed correlated with libido. Dennerstein has also found that young women who've had their ovaries surgically removed (for various reasons but often as part of cancer treatment), resulting in a sudden loss of oestrogen, also report lost libido.[157]

Further evidence for the role of oestrogen in promoting desire comes from reports that some women on the pill lose their sex drive – about fifteen per cent, according to a 2013 review.[158] This is potentially problematic for women who start taking the pill in their early teens. They may never have experienced strong sexual desire or arousal and, to put it bluntly, may not know what they're missing.

Let's talk about sexual response cycles

Of course, there's far more to our complex and nuanced sex lives than hormones and fertility. Sometimes we're wildly turned on by a mere thought. Other times even the most skilled attention by a romantic partner leaves us cold. Sometimes we're horny as anything when the chance of pregnancy is nil. Sometimes we desire sex during our periods, when we're pregnant, after menopause and with other women. We have sex for all sorts of reasons and getting pregnant isn't usually the end goal. One survey of 3000 men and women identified no less than 237 different reasons for wanting to have sex![159]

To understand how our minds, bodies and brains process hundreds of reasons why, it's worth understanding the so-called sexual response cycle. The basic phases of the sexual response cycle were first described back in the 1960s by pioneering sex researchers William Masters and Virginia Johnson. Their four-step model based on '10 000 complete cycles of sexual response' was linear and assumed men and women progressed sequentially through each phase: arousal, plateau, orgasm and finally to resolution or satisfaction.

As you'd expect, the basic model has been challenged and refined over the years.

The first challenge was made by sex educator Beverly Whipple, who pointed out that some women move from arousal to orgasm without ever experiencing desire, or may experience arousal and satisfaction without climaxing.[160, 161] Another researcher, Rosemary Basson, proposed an alternative circular model which incorporates such things as a woman's need for intimacy, the fact that desire can be responsive or spontaneous, and desire may come either before or after physical arousal. Crucially, Basson's model considers the importance of the larger context of women's lives, in particular the relationship between the women and her partner.[161, 162] Another discovery calling the linear model into question was the finding that many women show a disconnect between their subjective arousal state

('I'm feeling turned on') and physiological measures of arousal (measures of vaginal lubrication or congestion). Men's responses are rarely disconnected. Erections and arousal are tightly linked and boys figure this out pretty early on in puberty.

And, of course, let's not ignore the contributions made by lab rodents who've helped us understand the neurobiology. In rodents, the phases of sexual pleasure – excitement, plateau, orgasm and refraction – adhere very well to other 'pleasure cycles' such as hunger or thirst. Basically, rodents have shown us we want something (motivation), like something (pleasure), have our fill (satiety) and either stick around for more or move on. I acknowledge that neuroscience removes a little of the romantic frisson.

Turning on the 'ONs' and turning off the 'OFFs'

My favourite researcher in female sexuality, Emily Nagoski, a sex educator and author of *Come As You Are* and the delightful TEDx talk 'Unlocking the Door to Your Authentic Sexual Wellbeing', does an impressive job weaving numerous threads into a coherent story.

Nagoski explains that our desire results from a balance between 'ON' and 'OFF' mechanisms in the brain. According to the dual-control model, an 'accelerator' notices all the sexually relevant information that might turn you on, whereas the 'brakes' notice all the reasons not to turn on. Thus, the process of becoming aroused involves both 'turning on the "ONs"' *and* 'turning off the "OFFs"'. 'Your level of sexual arousal at any given moment is the product of how much stimulation the accelerator is getting and how little stimulation the brakes are getting,' explains Nagoski.[163]

According to Nagoski, if you're struggling to get aroused, you might be suffering from lack of accelerator, a highly sensitive brake, or a bit of both. It turns out some difficulties with arousal can be solved by pushing harder on the accelerator; however, sensitive brakes are the stronger predictor of sexual problems. Nagoski suggests that if you're a woman who has trouble having an orgasm or takes an hour to get there, you may take a lot of 'ON' activity to generate a really high level of sexual tension, and a tiny touch of anxiety or stress to hit your brakes. Because orgasms happen when you generate a sufficient level of sexual tension in your body to cross a threshold, she suggests using a vibrator to learn how to climax. Essentially the vibrator floors the accelerator and overrides the brakes.

Cleverly, the dual-control model conceptualises sexual excitation and inhibition as separate systems. This is in contrast to the more traditional way of thinking about arousal as a linear process. The beauty of the dual-control model is that it recognises we're all different. What turns each of us on and off differs widely.

Where are the brain's ON and OFF switches?

The dual-control system is theoretical. As yet, there are no precisely identified ON or OFF switches in the brain. Just think of all the sensations, thoughts and feelings that can turn you on or off: feeling loved, novelty, potential pregnancy, how you feel about your body, how you feel about how your partner feels about your body, your trauma history, tiredness, the grocery list. Clearly, integrating this information requires multiple brain networks.

Sexual excitation probably involves brain networks utilising the neurochemicals dopamine, oxytocin, vasopressin and noradrenaline. We know dopamine release leads to feelings of intense pleasure (liking) and the motivation to seek out the pleasurable experience again (wanting). Interestingly, a well-documented side effect of Parkinson's disease treatment, whereby dopamine levels are increased with drugs, is enhanced libido. And looping back to the role of hormones, oestrogen facilitates dopamine release, perhaps accounting for the experience of 'wanting' or desire around ovulation.[164]

Sexual inhibition likely involves the same brain networks as arousal; however, activity may be dampened by serotonin and the endocannabinoid systems. These brain chemicals are involved in sexual satiety and the refractory period after orgasm.[165, 166]

One of the strongest lines of evidence implicating serotonin in sexual braking is the effect antidepressants, especially SSRIs, have on sexual responses. One side effect of SSRIs is the inability to achieve orgasm. In fact, the strong braking effect of SSRIs has resulted in their off-label use to treat premature ejaculation. Serotonin is generally inhibitory to sexual responses in rats too. Male rats allowed to mate until they're sexually exhausted can be encouraged to respond to the solicitations of females if they're injected with drugs that block serotonin. Female rats given SSRIs tend to steer clear of male rats, and reduce the amount of time they display lordosis when they're fertile.

Can drugs be used to hit the sexual accelerator or brake?

If drugs that increase serotonin dampen desire, and drugs that increase dopamine can potentially fire up arousal, why not simply pop a pill to 'turn on the ONs' and 'turn off the OFFs'?

Drugs that selectively activate the accelerator or release the brakes are in use to treat hypoactive sexual desire disorder (HSDD), a type of sexual dysfunction affecting approximately ten per cent of adult women. HSDD is characterised by loss of desire and, importantly, is accompanied by frustration, grief, sadness, or worry concerning the lost libido.[165] One such drug used to treat HSDD is flibanserin (sold under the brand name Addyi and sometimes known as 'pink viagra'). Flibanserin is currently approved to treat HSDD by the United States Food and Drug Administration (US FDA), but is not yet available in many countries, including Australia.

Flibanserin works by increasing dopamine and decreasing serotonin. In other words, it's perfectly designed to simultaneously hit the accelerator and release the brakes.

When Addyi was first launched it was welcomed as a win by women's sexual health campaigners who for years had bemoaned the fact that men had Viagra and women had nothing. Other groups, however, have questioned whether libido can actually be fixed by a pill.[167] Looking at the data, it is easy to see where the scepticism comes from. Compared to a placebo, women taking Addyi reported only one more 'sexually satisfying event' per month accompanied by very little increase in actual desire. Or, put another way, women taking Addyi have more frequent sex, but they don't 'want' it more often. Addyi also comes with significant side effects including low blood pressure, fainting, nausea and dizziness, all of which are heightened when women drink alcohol.

Testosterone – does it really boost libido in women?

In Australia, where flibanserin is not available, post-menopausal women are often prescribed testosterone to treat low desire. It has been known since the early 1940s that very high doses of testosterone increase arousal in women.

Professor Susan Davis, an endocrinologist and women's health specialist at Monash University, has prescribed testosterone for loss of interest in sex in women. She has found about sixty per cent of women suffering low libido respond well, twenty per cent don't respond at all, and for twenty per cent it makes things worse.[168]

Bear in mind that when it comes to sex, responding 'well' is a matter of opinion, and naturally menopausal women taking testosterone report an extra one to two 'sexually satisfying experiences' per month. Women who've experienced surgical menopause report in the order of two to three extra sexually satisfying experiences per month when taking high doses of testosterone compared to a placebo.[169]

Testosterone might be intimately entwined with arousal and desire in men, but its use in women remains controversial. First, no trial of testosterone has run for more than three years, so the long-term effects and risks of testosterone on women's health are unknown. Second, there is little evidence that testosterone itself predicts desire across the monthly cycle or after menopause. Third, testosterone doesn't appear to help low sex drive in *pre-*menopausal women.

How testosterone works to increase desire when it does 'work' remains yet another great unknown in the world of female brain research. Testosterone is converted to oestrogen in the brain, so it might work by increasing oestrogen levels towards those naturally occurring around ovulation.

The women's health organisation Jean Hailes for Women's Health states that the relationship between testosterone and libido is very complex and age, mood, general wellbeing, and the potential risks of testosterone therapy must be taken into account when making the choice whether to use it. Stress, relationships and emotions have far more influence on women's sexual desire, and as Susan Davis points out, if your relationship has gone sour, 'it can't be fixed with hormones'.

The current best treatment for HSDD or low libido is the bio-psychosocial approach, that is, taking into account bottom-up, outside-in and top-down factors. Sex therapy teaches women how their sexuality is influenced by negative thoughts, beliefs, expectations, cultural and religious standards, moods and relationships (not just hormones!), and how desire can be spontaneous and come from within (top-down from our thoughts) or from the outside world (from the touch of an attentive lover). By learning and practising a variety of exercises that attempt to improve awareness of the here and now, acceptance and self-compassion, women often become 'more comfortable being in their own skin', sex therapist and sexologist Isiah McKimmie told me. 'Let's not forget, what's happening outside the bedroom influences what is happening inside the bedroom,' she said.

Mating in captivity – are you just bored?

McKimmie explained that the early honeymoon phase of a relationship is known as 'limerence' – that fantastical stage when you can't keep your hands off each other. Limerence typically fades after a few years when the reality of everyday life kicks in. 'It doesn't mean you're no longer in love, or don't care, it means you're entering a new phase,' she said. The trouble is, the 'death of eros' is often accompanied by loss of libido.

Here's an interesting twist to the story: loss of libido isn't so much about biology as it is about boredom, especially for midlife women in long-term relationships.

Dennerstein found that women who took a new lover after the menopause reported their libido to be unchanged by their 'ageing hormonal status'. Her 2002 Australian study tracked hundreds of women from their forties through menopause, and found dampened sexual enthusiasm was more closely related to long-term stale relationships than ageing ovaries. For women in new relationships limerence triumphed over hormonal factors.[157, 170] This result flies in the face of popular wisdom (and conventional couples therapy) that assumes women require security, familiarity and monogamy to feel sexual desire.

Daniel Bergner, author of *What Do Women Want? Adventures in the Science of Female Desire*, and Esther Perel, author of the delightfully titled *Mating in Captivity: Sex, Lies and Domestic Bliss*, both make compelling cases that the cause of lack of desire in women is boredom.[171, 172]

In her experience as a sex therapist, Perel believes that increased emotional intimacy is often accompanied by *decreased* desire. 'What makes for good intimacy does not always make for good sex,' she says. For some couples, good communication, mutual respect, and honesty are tightly correlated to an 'ongoing, pulsing erotic bond'. But for others the breakdown of desire is a consequence of the creation of intimacy. In her therapy practice, Perel counsels couples that the fundamental aspects of desire and yearning can be recreated within long-term relationships by injecting mystery, distance, and planning erotic 'other-than-vanilla' sex escapades. Daniel Bergner and his long-term girlfriend's solution to recapturing desire is more pragmatic: they now live six blocks apart.

Sexual orientation and the brain

Recently a colleague, University of Otago psychologist and author Jesse Bering, explained that gender is between the ears, sex is in the chromosomes and orientation is what turns you on – and that none of these are choices.

Bering's statement is backed up by extensive research on the biological factors influencing sexual orientation. As briefly outlined in the introduction to this book, all people have a sexual orientation that's separate from their biological sex and gender identity.

What does neuroscience have to say on the topic of sexual orientation? As yet, science can't fully explain how the brain generates various gender-related behaviours, sexual orientation or gender identity. 'The relative contributions of genetic determinants and social experience remain to be determined,' from *Principles of Neural Science* is a pretty typical statement in the literature.

However, it is widely acknowledged that sexual orientation is multi-dimensional and that for some people, especially women, it's dynamic and changes through the lifespan. The Dunedin Study found that same-sex attraction is more common among women than men at all ages.[173]

It's worth noting that the Dunedin cohort were born in the mid-1970s, and if we look to younger generations, many are rejecting typical gender and sexual norms, and recognising that sexual orientation and gender are fluid.[174] For example, The Massive Millennial Poll, a survey of 1000 people aged eighteen to thirty-four, found that over half believe gender is a spectrum and shouldn't be limited to the categories of male and female.[175]

Irrespective of your sexual orientation, being deeply in love with a man or a woman activates the same circuits in the brain. When Semir Zeki scanned the brains of twenty-four people, half of whom were female (six gay and six straight) and half male (six gay and six straight), while they viewed images of their sweethearts, the pattern of activation was the same in everyone. As Zeki points out, we didn't need neuroscience to tell us this. The world literature of love does not differentiate between gay, straight and otherwise. 'Indeed, the sentiments expressed are so similar as to introduce a profound ambiguity that makes it easy to read these texts in the opposite- or same-sex contexts, regardless of the authors' intentions,' writes Zeki. 'This is true of the sonnets of Shakespeare, among others, and is much aided where the language used is silent as to gender, as in the poetry of Rumi and Hafiz in Farsi.'[176] Love conquers all. #loveislove.

The neurobiology of orgasms

If you've figured out how to 'turn on the ONs' and 'turn off the OFFs', you've attracted a mate and decided to have sex, or you're taking matters into your own hands, what happens in your brain and nervous system as you become aroused and reach orgasm?

First, let's define 'orgasm'.

One current working definition states: 'An orgasm in the human female is a variable, transient peak sensation of intense pleasure, creating an altered state of consciousness, usually with an initiation accompanied by involuntary, rhythmic contractions of the pelvic striated circumvaginal musculature, often with concomitant uterine and anal contractions, and myotonia that resolves the sexually induced vasocongestion and myotonia, generally with an induction of well-being and contentment.' (Note, myotonia = muscle relaxation, vasocongestion = swelling of genitals with blood.)[177]

Emily Nagoski uses a simpler definition: 'Orgasm is a sudden, involuntary release of sexual tension.'

What are the neural pathways involved in the 'involuntary, rhythmic contractions' and 'release of sexual tension'?

Let's start with the clitoris, for it has no purpose other than generating female orgasms (the stats back this up, with the Kinsey Institute reporting eighty to ninety per cent of women who masturbate reach orgasm via clitoris stimulation alone).

Not unlike an iceberg, ninety per cent of the clitoris lies hidden beneath the surface of the vulva. Given the lack of attention paid to female health, it is hardly surprising a comprehensive account of clitoral anatomy was not provided until 2005, when Australian urologist Helen O'Connell published her *Journal of Urology* paper 'Anatomy of the Clitoris'. Using MRI, anatomical dissections and an extensive review of the current and historical literature, O'Connell gave us our first detailed description of clitoral anatomy, blood and nervous supply. In her paper, she pointed out that as recently as 1999 anatomy textbooks omitted a description of the clitoris. By comparison it would be hard to find an anatomy text from any period of history that omitted the penis.[178]

Now we understand that the clitoris is a multi-part system made up of the clitoral shaft, the crura or internal 'legs' of the clitoris, the corpus carvernosum, the urethral sponge and the vestibular bulbs on the inside. If you're having trouble visualising it, it's shaped rather like a wishbone with legs wrapping down around the urethra and vagina (or, as I've heard described, 'a neck travel pillow').

The pudendal nerve, derived from the Latin word *pudenda* (meaning 'the shameful parts'), innervates the clitoris, and the skin and muscles of the anus, perineum and pelvis. The pudendal nerve is actually a pair of nerves, one for each side of the pelvis, that has a complex anatomy with intricate branching patterns. It's not uncommon for the nerve to become injured during a difficult birth, sometimes leaving untreated women incontinent, with perineal pain and sexual dysfunction. Neurons from the pudendal nerve arise from a structure in the spinal cord called Onuf's nucleus, one of the few truly sexually dimorphic structures in the nervous system – it's much larger in males than females because it contains more cells. At the same time, it's widely reported that there are twice as many nerve endings in the clitoris compared to the head of the penis (8000 versus 4000) – I've been unable to find any academic literature to support or refute this claim.

The shameful nerve should stand proud, as it's the only nerve in the human body containing three neural sub-types: sensory neurons, motor neurons and autonomic neurons. Touch your clitoris and you'll trigger signals that will travel along sensory neurons into the spinal cord and up to your brain. Practise squeezing your pelvic floor muscles (also called 'Kegel exercises') and the muscle contractions will be initiated by signals travelling down the motor neurons of the pudendal nerve. Experience the involuntary rhythmic contractions of orgasm – they come about via signals transmitted along the sympathetic neurons of the pudendal nerve.

Of course, reaching orgasm is more complicated than triggering spinal reflexes. When the clitoris is fondled in just the right way, sensory neurons relay the signal to the spinal cord (the circuit sends another signal back to the genitals to increase blood flow and lubrication) and signals are relayed up to sexual centres in the brain, including those in the hypothalamus, hippocampus, amygdala, thalamus and cerebellum. There signals are modified as they integrate with visual cues, sounds, smells, thoughts and memories – ultimately, the ONs get turned on and the OFFs off, leading to the sensation of orgasm.

This is her brain during orgasm

Researchers have been observing and documenting our physiological sexual responses – blood pressure, heart rate, vaginal lubrication and so on – since the days of Alfred Kinsey, Masters and Johnson. But only in recent years, with the advent of modern brain-scanning technology, have we been able to observe what is happening in the brain in real time when we climax.

Kayt Sukel, author of the book *This is Your Brain on Sex*, is possibly better known as the woman who masturbated in an fMRI scanner so the world could watch her brain orgasm. Sukel did the deed in the Rutgers University research lab of Barry Komisaruk, watched over by then postdoctoral research fellow Nan Wise. In her book Sukel gives an entertaining account of the process, including descriptions of practising at home with a bell taped to her forehead as she learned to pleasure herself without moving (remaining completely still is essential for fMRI).

No less than thirty discrete brain areas were activated before, during and after Sukel's orgasm. A description of the patterns of brain activity in the *Guardian* newspaper mentions how activity first builds in the genital area of the sensory cortex then spreads to the limbic system (involved in emotion and memory).

> The orgasm arrives, activity shoots up in two parts of the brain called the cerebellum and the frontal cortex, perhaps because of greater muscle tension. During orgasm, activity reaches a peak in the hypothalamus, which releases a chemical called oxytocin that causes pleasurable sensations and stimulates the uterus to contract. Activity also peaks in the nucleus accumbens, an area linked to reward and pleasure. After orgasm, the activity in all these regions gradually calms down.[179]

Upon viewing Sukel's fMRI, Nan Wise observed, 'An orgasm really is a whole-brain kind of experience.' Wise, who also 'donates' her orgasms in the name of neuroscience, and says she hopes her research will eventually address gaps in the scientific literature regarding the neural basis of human sexuality. Right there is another PhD project waiting patiently for attention.

The neurobiology of multiple orgasms

Time and time again while writing this book I've set out to research a particular topic expecting to find plenty of neuroscience literature, only to discover another gaping hole in our knowledge. While multiple orgasms are well described in the sexual health literature, like the clitoris they're mysteriously missing from biology texts.

One PubMed search I ran found only five reviews on multiple orgasms, three of which are about men, not women. One paper titled 'Multiple Orgasms in Men–What We Know So Far' concluded, 'Despite popular interest, the topic of male multiple orgasms has received surprisingly little scientific assessment.' Substitute 'female' in place of 'male' and the sentence retains accuracy. I asked researcher Brendan Zietsch (who has written academic articles about the female orgasm) if there was some literature I'd simply missed. He confirmed my findings – or lack thereof. Most of the literature focuses on women who never reach orgasm (anorgasmia) or who find it very difficult to climax (about one in ten women never have orgasms, and about one third struggle to climax regularly).[180]

The best the academic literature can provide is to state that men don't have multiple orgasms because they experience a 'latent state of arousal' or 'refractory period' after ejaculation. The male refractory period can last for minutes (in teenage boys) to days (in older men), but the reasons why are obscure. From a brain perspective, after ejaculation prolactin levels rise and dopamine and testosterone levels plummet, dampening sexual desire and arousal. One suggestion is that it gives time for sperm to be produced again, and prevents the displacement of previously ejaculated sperm. It might also protect men from overstimulating their penis, resulting in irritation, and help men avoid physical exhaustion. Presumably, the same refractory period doesn't exist in women. Aren't we lucky!

A Finnish survey gives an insight into the characteristics of multi-orgasmic women.[180]

- ♀ About one in ten women had two or more orgasms in their latest intercourse.
- ♀ Women who regularly experience multiple orgasms considered orgasm in intercourse as 'very important'.
- ♀ Multi-orgasmic women displayed strong sexual interests, and were sexually very active often, regularly used sex toys, and engaged in daily sexual intercourse.
- ♀ Multi-orgasmic women achieved frequent orgasms just as easily via masturbation as love-making.

The authors couldn't conclude whether experiencing joy during sex resulted in these women being multi-orgasmic, or if it is a case of the very positive sexual experiences encouraging sexual appetites.

Are female orgasms just a happy accident?

Unlike the male orgasm, which is the reward that comes from depositing one's sperm, female orgasms are unnecessary for conception. So why do we experience them at all?

Numerous ideas persist among those who ponder such issues (upwards of twenty-one theories, according to Elisabeth Lloyd, who wrote an entire book, *The Case of the Female Orgasm: Bias in the Science of Evolution*, examining each idea). Some theories consider the female orgasm to be an evolutionary adaptation necessary for promoting pair bonding. When we orgasm, concentrations of arousing neurotransmitters flood our body and brain, promoting feelings of connection and emotional closeness. If your partner makes you feel good then you're more likely to stay together to raise any offspring.[181]

Another school of thought proposes that during orgasm the cervix rhythmically dips up and down into the pool of semen (presumably already left behind) and sucks sperm into the uterus, thereby increasing the probability of conception. The 'in-suck theory' (their words, not mine) has been extensively studied using a variety of technologies, including tiny penis-mounted cameras in humans. But results are conflicting. One recent study found there was a significant difference in semen retention when women orgasmed, but it wasn't linked to improved fertility.[182]

The current favoured philosophy is the 'happy accident' that suggests orgasms are a by-product (or fantastic bonus, depending on how you see it) of early embryonic development whereby the male and female genitalia arise from the same tissue. Some liken the clitoris to a tiny vestigial penis that just happens to provide orgasms to females only because they're necessary for males to achieve reproductive success. In other words, we have orgasms by default (or perhaps destiny).[182]

Can we become addicted to love?

Love researchers suggest that the symptoms of falling in love and into addiction are very similar. New lovers, like all addicts, yearn for their new love (craving); they feel a rush of exhilaration when seeing or thinking about him or her (euphoria/intoxication) and seek to interact with their beloved more and more frequently over time (tolerance). Then, like addicts, if the relationship sours, the common signs of withdrawal set in: crying, lethargy, anxiety, insomnia and so on. 'Like most addicts, rejected lovers also often go to extremes, even sometimes doing degrading or physically dangerous things to win back the beloved,' says Fisher.[183, 184]

Addictive substances hijack the dopamine pathways involved in motivation. Often called the 'pleasure' molecule, dopamine encourages 'wanting' more than 'liking'. Regardless of the stimulus, Fisher suspects our brains become habituated to elevated levels of dopamine, which is why the ecstasy of early romantic love doesn't last forever. If the 'liking' isn't there once the 'wanting' fades, people set off in search of the next rush. In her studies of people who remain happily in love and together after decades, a second neural network is recruited as true 'liking' sets in. This network is associated with attachment, empathy and emotional regulation. It turns out the deeply committed couples who remain in love not only continue to 'want' their partner, they quite like them too.[185]

Oxytocin – one molecule to love and bond us all?

To say we're social animals is a cliché, but from the moment we're born we're bound to others. 'Love is deeply biological,' write husband-and-wife team Sue Carter and Stephen Porges in *EMBO Reports*. 'It pervades every aspect of our lives and has inspired countless works of art. Love also has a profound effect on our mental and physical state.'[186]

When biologists dissect the biochemistry of love, they return time and time again to one molecule: oxytocin.

It wasn't that long ago that our interest in oxytocin was confined to its perfunctory roles in labour and lactation. Oxytocin is a neuropeptide (a small protein used by neurons to communicate) and it was originally extracted from puréed pituitary gland. In the early 1900s, British pharmacologist Henry Dale found he could hasten the labour of pregnant cats by injecting them with the pituitary extract. Within a couple of years, Dale's 'hormone of swift birth' was being administered to women in labour. Synthetic oxytocin is still used in labour wards today.

Oxytocin is released during labour and also causes the smooth muscle contractions responsible for milk let-down during breastfeeding. Oxytocin and the hormone prostaglandin are responsible for uterine contractions during the third stage of labour when the placenta is expelled. This is one reason why newborns are encouraged to breastfeed immediately after birth – oxytocin released by suckling encourages contractions to shrink the womb and reduce post-partum haemorrhage. And, handily, oxytocin compels mothers to nurture their babies and keep them close.

The effect of oxytocin on the mother–baby bond is seen to full effect in rodents. Normally a mother rat is very protective over her young and displays stereotypical maternal behaviours: she keeps her pups clustered together in a group, crouches over them, licks them, builds a nest, and if one pup becomes separated she'll scurry over and drag the pup back to the litter. Neuroendocrinologists have discovered that infusing oxytocin into the brains of virgin rats causes them to behave as if they are the loving birth mothers to foster pups.[187]

If oxytocin was responsible for the kisses and cuddles I smothered my boys with after the agony and exhaustion of giving birth, it gets plenty of respect from me.

Oxytocin – what we've learned from the monogamous prairie vole

Oxytocin isn't only the purveyor of the bond between mother and child, it also promotes male and female bonding after mating (and, presumably, more so after orgasm).

We've learned much of what we know about oxytocin and pair-bonding from prairie voles. They're the darlings of oxytocin research, because unlike most rodents – which have a deserved reputation for promiscuity – prairie voles are monogamous and mate for life. Sue Carter, the grand dame of oxytocin researchers, has spent her career studying prairie voles and has found that oxytocin together with its sister neuropeptide, vasopressin, underly vole devotion.

Oxytocin and vasopressin are synthesised by neurons in the hypothalamus. The two neuropeptides are then transported along axons directly to the pituitary gland, where they're packaged into vesicles and stored for release into the bloodstream as hormones. Oxytocin and vasopressin also act as neurotransmitters. Oxytocin- and vasopressin-containing neurons project from the hypothalamus to brain regions involved in social and emotional processing, such as the amygdala, hippocampus and nucleus accumbens.

Oxytocin and vasopressin are released during mating. They reduce fear and anxiety by decreasing amygdala activity – a key region in the brain's fear network – and they support lordosis. Oxytocin, especially, lowers the natural resistance most animals have to the proximity of others, facilitating what are known as 'approach behaviours'. It goes without saying that you need to get in quite close proximity to another of your species to procreate.

Compared to their promiscuous cousins, prairie voles have higher levels of oxytocin and more receptors for the neuropeptide in their brains. If oxytocin release is blocked, prairie voles act like typical rodents – they have fleeting episodes of mating and don't settle down with one partner for life. Some very clever scientists have genetically manipulated the brains of mice to express prairie-vole-like patterns of oxytocin, which causes mice to behave much more like their monogamous cousins.

Oxytocin, working in concert with a host of neurochemicals, has been implicated in an extraordinary number of social behaviours and physiological roles. A non-comprehensive taster list of oxytocin actions includes:

- ♀ Suppresses stress hormones cortisol and noradrenaline, and slows heart rate.
- ♀ Facilitates paternal care.
- ♀ Modulates distress in pups separated from their mother.
- ♀ Decreases anxiety and depression via oestrogen signalling.
- ♀ Is important for foetal heart development, and in adults protects against heart disease.
- ♀ Accelerates adult neurogenesis (in rodents).[186, 188, 189]

Looking at this list, it's easy to see why we get excited by the human potential contained in one tiny molecule (or two, if you include vasopressin). However, like all signalling pathways connecting body and brain, oxytocin and vasopressin can only exert their effect by 'locking in' to their receptors. And like all receptors, oxytocin and vasopressin receptors are regulated by genes, hormones, epigenetic factors and life experiences. It's never quite as simple as we would like.

Social support buffers stress because of oxytocin

In her TED talk, 'How to make stress your friend', psychologist Kelly McGonigal proposes that oxytocin nudges you to share your feelings when you're stressed. 'When life is difficult, your stress response wants you to be surrounded by people who care about you,' she says.[190]

We've explored the concept of social buffering throughout this book – it occurs not only for the mother–infant relationship but also in adult relationships, and time and again we've seen how social support and love vaccinate against stress. Oxytocin may be the missing link.

It turns out that oxytocin is released not only in response to positive social interactions but to very stressful experiences too (well, at least this is the case in rodents – we don't yet know if this occurs in humans). Oxytocin modulates the HPA axis and immune system. In both animals and humans, injecting oxytocin lowers blood levels of cortisol. 'The protective effects of positive sociality seem to rely on the same cocktail of hormones that carry a biological message of "love" throughout the body,' writes Sue Carter. 'The same molecules that allow us to give and receive love, also link our need for others with health and well-being.'[186]

At the same time as having a physiological effect on our stress response, oxytocin works to counter stress by 'nudging' people to seek support, in turn upping oxytocin levels further. It's been suggested that the very strong emotional bonds that form between folk during periods of extreme duress, especially when the survival depends on the presence and support of others, are due to oxytocin.

As McGonigal says, 'When you choose to connect with others under stress you can create resilience.'

Is oxytocin the new love potion?

Untangling oxytocin's role in humans is clearly going to be more challenging than in prairie voles. Oxytocin is not the molecular *equivalent* of love – it's just one important component of a neurochemical system that allows us to respond emotionally to others.

Despite the cautiousness of biologists, oxytocin has earned a global reputation as the molecule of love and cuddles, trust, intimacy and the molecule that binds tribes. A quick online search confirms oxytocin's potential. 'Oxytocin: could the "trust hormone" rebond our troubled world?' asks one headline. 'The Moral Molecule: How oxytocin can revolutionise your organisation', says another. Recently I read an article that gave an explanation why my cocker spaniel is so overly friendly and clingy: oxytocin.

One classic study published in *Nature* in 2005 found that people given sniffs of oxytocin were more willing to entrust large sums of money to strangers in a role-playing investment game. The authors concluded (in rather an overstatement) that oxytocin is essential for trust and the normal operation of human societies, and that oxytocin 'contributes to economic, political and social success'.[191] A commentary by neuroscientist Antonio Damasio raised the disturbing prospect that the findings may result in political operators generously spraying crowds at their rallies with oxytocin. Before you fret too much about this notion, five subsequent studies failed to replicate the original 2005 findings.[192]

The hype surrounding oxytocin has led to online retailers selling bottles of the stuff in attractively packaged glass spray bottles – 'Connekt' in blue for him, and 'Attrakt' in pink for her. 'Better Together!'

As you can imagine, such marketing spin results in plenty of neuroendocrinologists' foreheads being banged on lab benches round the world.

One problem with all human studies is that we don't know if oxytocin sprayed up the nose enters the brain. And if it does, does it reach oxytocin receptor sites? We understand that neuropeptides can travel in one direction only, from brain to body, and not the other way round. Unlike fat-soluble hormones such as oestrogen or testosterone, oxytocin and vasopressin cannot cross the blood–brain barrier. Some claim nasal sprays sidestep the blood–brain barrier; others argue we have no firm evidence.[188]

Naturally occurring oxytocin has some surprisingly negative emotional effects too. Women who breastfeed display a 'mama bear' effect whereby they show more aggression when threatened. And oxytocin increases envy, gloating and anger, which, to be fair, are all approach behaviours. Anger focuses your attention towards the target of your anger, as does envy. It's not all love and cuddles – even the love molecule has a dark, immoral side.[193]

Carter and others are particularly concerned by reports that state children with autism and adults with schizophrenia are being treated with oxytocin off-label. We have no evidence that autism or schizophrenia are affected by levels of oxytocin.[188]

'We do not understand how the hormone works yet, or have enough information about what happens when it's given repeatedly,' Carter says in an interview with *Nature*. 'This is not a molecule that people should be self-administering or playing with.'[194]

At our wedding, my husband and I danced to Blur's 'Tender'. The song claims that love is the greatest thing that we have. Indeed, love is great, complex, mysterious – and more magnificent than a single molecule.

8.

Pregnancy and Motherhood

MOTHERHOOD IS THE BEGINNING OF ONE OF LIFE'S GREAT LOVE stories. It recalibrates our course and realigns our lives.

This book is dedicated to my boys, Harry and Jamie, for good reason. Yes, I realise it is the ultimate cliché, but becoming their mother changed everything. Having children threw the pieces of my life up in the air. The pieces settled again, but my body, outlook on life, sense of self and emotions have never been quite the same. Not only did I birth two beautiful boys into the world, I birthed a new identity as a mother.

My experience is not unique. For those who are mothers it's one of the most fundamental transformations we go through as women. For many of us, parenthood brings with it identity changes and conflicting emotions: love, protectiveness, joy, nurturing, exhaustion, confusion, anger and apathy.

During pregnancy, a cocktail of hormones prepares your body for birth and breastfeeding. You grow an entirely new organ, the placenta, to ensure your baby receives nutrients and to buffer her against stress. Your metabolism resets to store energy for foetal development and lactation. Your breasts grow so you can nurse. Once your baby arrives, she's so irresistible you become consumed by her, and spend much of your time caressing, holding, feeding, gazing at her and breathing in her scent. These maternal behaviours, as they're called, are essential for the survival of your newborn.

The same hormonal cocktail profoundly alters the architecture of your brain, in particular structures underlying social cognition and emotion. These brain changes last, and the changes in the brains and behaviours of mothers are evident throughout the lifespan.

So, here's a new way to think about pregnancy – changes to your *body* ensure your baby is carried safely to term; and changes to your *brain* ensure you're prepared for the social and emotional challenges of motherhood.

Elsewhere we've focused on how parenting influences child development; here we'll flip that picture and look at how children wield remarkable influence over their mother's brain. Mother Nature may be a driving force during pregnancy, but the experience of nurturing comes to the fore after birth. Maternal behaviours are partly the product of the maternal brain networks that have been primed by the hormones of pregnancy and childbirth, but such behaviours are refined and reinforced by the experience of parenthood itself.

In the pages that follow, I'll take you on a tour of pregnancy, childbirth and the early stages of motherhood. Indeed, pregnancy and motherhood are accompanied by some of the most dramatic plasticity the female brain undergoes during life.

Pregnancy leads to long-lasting changes in women's brains

A paper published in December 2016 in *Nature Neuroscience* gave us our first detailed insight into how pregnancy changes the structure of women's brains. Using MRI, a team of researchers led by Elseline Hoekzema scanned the brains of twenty-five first-time mothers before and after pregnancy, and compared their brains to twenty women who'd never been pregnant.[195]

Pregnancy was associated with pronounced and long-lasting grey matter *shrinkage* in regions of the cortex related to social cognition, empathy and theory of mind. The hippocampus, a region associated with memory, also lost volume.

The grey matter changes induced by pregnancy were anything but subtle. Notably, a computer program was able to automatically determine whether or not a woman had undergone pregnancy based only on her brain scans.

Some of the brain changes were long lasting. Two years after the initial scan, eleven of the women who hadn't fallen pregnant for a second time were invited back and their brains scanned again. In all women, the cortical alterations had endured, but the hippocampus recovered volume.

In some ways, the plastic changes are not dissimilar to those seen in adolescence when pubertal hormones trigger thinning of the PFC. It's likely that a similar process of refinement and specialisation of the social brain is taking place during pregnancy. As I discussed in chapters 2 and 5, *loss* of grey matter volume reflects synaptic pruning and 'functional streamlining' of circuits, not degeneration.

Because the grey matter changes occurred in regions associated with theory of mind networks, Hoekzema ran a series of tests to see if changes were related to real-life skills. The first was a survey of maternal attachment, which included statements such as 'I would describe my feelings for the baby as dislike' or 'intense affection', or 'When I have to leave the baby: I usually feel rather sad' or 'rather relieved'. The greater the strength of the bonding between a mother and her baby, the greater the degree of grey matter plasticity.

Theory of mind is linked to the ability to read faces and emotions. An fMRI scan monitored the mother's brain responses to photos of either their own or strangers' babies. When women looked at photos of their own little bundles, regions that showed the strongest neural activation corresponded to the regions that thinned during pregnancy. Looking at a baby other than their own had no effect on neural activity. This supported the idea that brain plasticity occurred in areas linked to social cognition, empathy and theory of mind.

In rodents, the hippocampus is one of only a few brain regions to show neurogenesis throughout adulthood. During pregnancy and lactation, neurogenesis slows then recovers again after weaning. A similar process may account for the shrinkage and subsequent recovery of the hippocampus in women. Because the hippocampus is involved in memory, the team speculated that grey matter loss may be related to the memory problems some women report during pregnancy (known colloquially as 'pregnancy brain' or 'baby brain'). Hoekzema thus conducted a series of verbal and short-term memory tests to see if women's memory loss was due to hippocampal shrinkage. However, they found no memory changes during or after pregnancy.

The process of becoming a parent for the first time is an intense, all-encompassing experience, so the obvious question to ask is whether it's pregnancy and childbirth or the experience of caring for a baby that tinkers with brain structure? The team tested for the effects of parenting versus pregnancy in a rather ingenious way. They scanned the brains of first-time *fathers* before and after their wives' pregnancies. No alterations in structure were observed in men's brains once they took on dad duties, which strongly suggests the women's brains were changed by pregnancy not parenting.

One of the strengths of this study was how thorough the researchers were. In case you're curious whether method of conception, delivery or feeding influenced brain structure (we're all partial to 'me-search re-search'), here are a few more details. Of the twenty-five women (average age thirty-four), nine achieved pregnancy by natural conception and sixteen used fertility treatment. Natural versus assisted conception had no impact on brain structure. Ten of the women had boys, eleven had girls, and four had twins (two mixed twins, one male twins, one female twins); the baby's sex had no effect on its mother's brain. Eight of the women gave birth by Caesarean section and seventeen by vaginal birth; style of delivery had no impact on the brain. Finally, most women exclusively breastfed, two breastfed and supplemented with formula, and four exclusively bottlefed (all babies were fed!); method of feeding had no effect on women's brain structure.

It's important to note that this study does not imply fathers nor non-birth mothers lack 'parenting brain circuitry' or a 'theory of mind', and it certainly does not let dads off the hook from parenting! But we don't need neuroscience to support or deny that fact anyway. Babies need warm, secure attachment with at least one parent to organise and regulate healthy brain development. Clearly a birth mother is not the only adult capable of being such a caregiver.

So, what is it about pregnancy that sculpts women's brains?

Hoekzema and colleagues propose it is 'the unequaled surges of sex steroid hormones that a woman is exposed to during her pregnancy'. Dramatic fluctuations in oestrogen, progesterone, prolactin, oxytocin and cortisol may drive synaptic pruning, gliogenesis or myelination. But MRI doesn't have the resolution to tell us this detail. Instead we need to turn our attention to the expectant brains of rodents.

The expectant rodent brain

Clearly, female rodents can't read books to find out what to expect when they're expecting; therefore, changes in how rodent mothers think, feel and behave must be driven entirely by biology. Kelly Lambert and Craig Kingsley, behavioural neuroscientists who study the neurobiology of parenting, say, 'The maternal brain is both the goal of the endocrine tsunami that accompanies pregnancy, and the culmination of millennia of natural selective processes.'

Pregnancy and motherhood change everything for rodents too. After giving birth, previously aloof female rats are transformed into attentive, nest-building, pup-grooming, nursing mamas. Because they don't have the luxury of learning how to parent, pregnancy hormones must prime their brains to mother. At birth, pups *and* maternal behaviours emerge simultaneously, and over subsequent days the same maternal behaviours are reinforced by experience – the sight, smell and sounds of the pups themselves.

Motherhood makes female rodents smarter. Compared to their child-free sisters, mothers are superior at learning, memory, foraging and predatory tasks. They're braver, less anxious and less stressed, but more aggressive when their brood is threatened. Once pups are weaned and females are faced with an empty nest, their newly acquired smarts persist for life. Older female rats who've had multiple pregnancies have better memories and show fewer signs of brain ageing than virgin sisters.[196]

The emergence of maternal behaviours and superior cognitive abilities in rodents has been neatly mapped onto 'maternal circuitry', the hub of which is the medial preoptic area (MPOA) of the hypothalamus. During labour, the sudden flood of oxytocin acts on receptors in the MPOA to ensure the maternal behaviours emerge at the same time as the pups. The MPOA is connected to brain regions involved in reward and motivation, which use the 'feel-good' neurotransmitter, dopamine (perhaps suggesting motherhood is, or should be, inherently rewarding).

The hippocampus – critical for memory formation, mood regulation and navigation – and the olfactory bulbs, critical for smell, also undergo plastic change during pregnancy, childbirth and lactation, including alterations in neuron number, neuro-chemistry and gene expression.[197]

Another type of plasticity involves dendritic spines – the tiny buds on dendrites on which synapses form. The growth and loss of spines reflects the formation and elimination of synapses. During pregnancy, spines flourish as if they've been fertilised by the hormonal milieu. Oestrogen is a potent modulator of spine dynamics, typically, the more oestrogen available, the more spines grow.

Do human mothers share the same maternal brain circuitry as other mammals?

We suspect so. For example, brain scans of brand new human mothers listening to their babies' cries show the hypothalamus and reward pathways are activated. And Hoekzema showed that human mothers' hippocampi change in size during pregnancy. But the big difference between humans and other animals is the involvement of our social brain.

As the saying goes, 'Nothing in biology makes sense except in light of evolution', and plasticity of the rodent maternal brain is critical because pup survival depends so heavily on a mother's ability to forage for food. Humans evolved under very different pressures, with foraging a less essential survival skill for the new human mum. Traditionally, we lived in large family groups and raised our children under the watchful eye of more experienced mothers and grandmothers. Fathers, siblings and cousins foraged and hunted for food, and other lactating mothers could supplement breastmilk. This legacy of 'alloparenting' has driven the evolution of our social brains, and is thought to drive plasticity and refinement of social brain networks during pregnancy.[198]

In researching this section of the book, I've spent countless hours reading blogs, articles and books on the topic of motherhood (clearly my own identity as a mother and woman is still top of mind). Again, one theme emerged as core to maternal wellbeing – love and social connection. It's often said it 'takes a village to raise a child', and the 'village' is missing from the lives of so many of today's modern women. I suspect, for some of us, motherhood is as solitary an activity as it is for the new rodent mother.[198]

Your expectant brain and hormones of pregnancy

When we first met the placenta back in chapter 1, I told you that this remarkable organ acts as an interface between a mother and her baby, moving oxygen, carbon dioxide, nutrients and waste; and as a buffer, selectively protecting the baby as much as possible from her mother's hormones and environmental stressors. The placenta also acts as a giant gland orchestrating the transition to motherhood.[199]

Immediately after implantation, the blastocyst (fertilised egg) starts producing hCG (giving you the longed-for, or feared, thin blue line on a positive pregnancy test). During the earliest stages of pregnancy, hCG maintains the corpus luteum, which develops in the ovary from a burst follicle. Although the exact reasons for the morning sickness that seventy to eighty per cent of women suffer in their first trimester are unknown, hCG usually takes the blame.

Under direct control from the foetus and placenta, the corpus luteum produces progesterone, literally the 'pro-gestation' hormone. Among other roles, progesterone suppresses the uterus's ability to contract, which protects against early labour, and suppresses fertility, preventing multiple differently timed pregnancies (can you just imagine?).

After a few months, when the ovaries become unable to keep up with endocrine demand, the placenta takes over manufacture of progesterone and oestrogen. Normally, ovarian progesterone and oestrogen levels are kept in check via HPO-axis feedback, but the placenta has no such constraints placed on it, so it floods the mother with hormones.

When you're pregnant, progesterone levels increase ten- to fifteen-fold. And oestrogen levels increase by 1000-fold, exceeding the *total* oestrogen exposure of the rest of your non-pregnant life. 'The foetus and placenta certainly make a loud orchestrated endocrine statement that they have arrived and intend to stay,' notes one neuroendocrinologist.[200]

As well as the flood of sex hormones, increased levels of neuropeptides (short protein molecules that act in the brain) flow into your bloodstream, including the two quintessential motherhood molecules: prolactin and oxytocin. Numerous other 'minor' placental hormones and molecules are produced, including growth hormone, kisspeptin, serotonin and relaxin, but for brevity in this chapter I'll focus on those that wield most influence over the female brain.

Prolactin – the quintessential hormone of pregnancy and parenting

Prolactin is a hormone that lacks the PR and newspaper headlines of its cuddly cousin oxytocin. Nonetheless, it has an unrivalled range of biological roles. First discovered and named because of its ability to promote milk production ('pro-lactation'), upwards of 300 roles have been identified, mostly related to pregnancy and motherhood.[201]

For this chapter I spoke to Dave Grattan, a professor of neuroendocrinology at the University of Otago in New Zealand. I got to know Grattan in 1996 when I was completing my undergraduate degree and he arrived at Otago to set up a new research group. Keeping it in the family, Grattan spent his early career working at the University of Maryland, where he collaborated with the doyenne of female brain development, Margaret McCarthy. Grattan calls prolactin '*the* quintessential pregnancy hormone' and over Skype he told me, 'Pregnancy, lactation and motherhood change every system in the body and brain, and for every change we've looked at so far, prolactin is involved.'

As a parenting hormone, prolactin is highly evolutionarily conserved. It is associated with brooding behaviour and nest-building in birds, and fin-fanning behaviour in some fish to induce fresh water flow over their eggs.[196] Mammals evolved after fish and birds, and it's thought prolactin was only co-opted as a lactation molecule later in evolution.

When we're not pregnant prolactin is produced by the anterior pituitary gland, but at only a trickle because it self-regulates its own secretion. During pregnancy, our remarkably plastic maternal brain switches 'off' the self-regulating feedback loop allowing for a sustained period of high prolactin secretion.[202]

During pregnancy, we require extra-high levels of prolactin and such levels can't be sustained by the pituitary alone, so the placenta makes its own version to top up supplies. Placental lactogen is molecularly identical to prolactin, and easily slips across the blood–brain barrier to latch onto prolactin receptors.[199, 202]

Prolactin, hunger and resisting the urge to eat for two

I felt prolactin's full effect in the first trimester of my first pregnancy when I developed a seriously insatiable hunger, tempered only by an extreme aversion to vegetables. My appetite was primal and overwhelming, and I was gripped not so much by wanting to eat as needing to *feed*. I'm not a big breakfast person, but I'd easily knock back a couple of bowls of oats and bananas, only to be starving by 10 a.m. I imagine if I was a laboratory rodent I'd have been logged as 'extremely hyperphagic'.

Prolactin acts on hormones that regulate your sense of hunger and satiety (feeling full). Normally these hormones sensibly signal when you're hungry or let you know when you've had your fill. In pregnancy, the signals are tipped towards eating more, which is Mother Nature's way of ensuring there are sufficient nutrients for the baby, sufficient energy for the extra metabolic strain on your body, and plenty of fat stores ready for breastfeeding.

Herein lies the rub. During early pregnancy, prolactin is signalling to you to eat more, slow down and store fat. But many women end up eating *significantly* more than is required to meet demand. This becomes a problem because some women (about half of pregnant women in Australia and New Zealand) are already overweight or obese at conception.

Weight gain in pregnancy is a combination of many factors – placenta, extra blood and amniotic fluid and, of course, the baby – not just fat stores. I was under the care of a doctor who believed in weighing his patients at every visit, and looking back at my antenatal data charts, prolactin clearly achieved its fat-accumulation targets – I put on more than half of my total additional pregnancy weight before week twelve.

Of course, your weight is not the sole indicator of health, but obesity at conception or gaining too much weight when you're pregnant is linked to increased risk for gestational diabetes, high blood pressure, pre-eclampsia, Caesarean section, and birth complications. Babies born to obese mothers are at risk of health problems such as heart disease and Type 2 diabetes in later life.[203, 204] Excessive weight gain often means that it is harder to lose weight after the baby is born (if bouncing back is your thing).

We're all different, but for a 'normal' healthy weight woman, the extra calories required during the first trimester can be met with a couple of extra pieces of fruit and half a glass of milk a day (the equivalent of one tiny unsatisfying snack, if you are anything like me). International guidelines give specific recommendations for pregnancy weight gain, but it won't surprise you to learn that we're not very good at following them.[205]

All this means is that the old-fashioned advice 'eat for two' – which made a lot of sense in the past when food was scarce – is not appropriate today. Instead, women are now warned to restrict their pregnancy weight gain, and the message has become, 'You're *not* eating for two', which for me confusingly translated to, 'Don't listen to your body.'

As Grattan points out, managing healthy weight gain, especially for those already overweight or obese, is pitting women against their biology. 'You're destined to fail because you're fighting an innate prolactin signal to eat and slow down,' said Grattan. 'At the same time this creates a very stressful situation, and we know excessive stress isn't good for any pregnancy.'

Pregnant women (like all people) should be entitled to receive evidence-based, compassionate and non-shaming care and advice. We all want to obtain optimal nutrition for our babies and ourselves, and weight loss or dieting is never encouraged during pregnancy. This is why weighing women at antenatal appointments is coming back into vogue – it opens the opportunity to chat about weight gain.

Clearly, *how* messages about weight gain and appetite management during pregnancy are delivered are as important as the messages themselves. I recall halfway through one of my pregnancies, working as a journalist at a medical conference, when a random doctor approached me during morning tea to say, 'You'll be more likely to have a vaginal birth if you put down that custard pastry.' Luckily for him, prolactin also acts to reduce stress levels and inhibit anxiety.

Pregnant women are less reactive to stress

As we learned in chapter 1, the nine months before we're born have the potential to shape the rest of our lives. Avoiding excess stress is important because cortisol pre-programs the infant's HPA axis, rendering her more reactive to stress and susceptible to poor health and mental illness as she grows up.

Pregnant women have developed in-built mechanisms to buffer babies against stress. As a first line of defence, our entire HPA axis quietens, which has a noteworthy side effect: we're less anxious and reactive to external stressors. As a second line of defence, the placenta contains an enzyme that converts the mother's cortisol to an inert steroid. However, the enzymatic barrier can be breached by infection, inflammation or excessive levels of maternal cortisol.

Because prolactin is the only hormonal signal that remains consistently elevated during pregnancy, it's the prime candidate for HPA-axis calming, lowered stress and anxiety.

In one experiment, researchers infused rats with prolactin and watched them explore a maze. Normally, non-pregnant rats are pretty anxious and aren't keen on exploring novel environments. Those infused with prolactin became very brave. They spent far more time than usual exploring and behaved like their adventurous pregnant sisters. In another test, rats took part in a ten-minute 'swimming test'. Rats don't like water but they're able to swim well and the swimming test is an established method for measuring rodent anxiety. When rats were infused with prolactin they didn't give up and float around helplessly in the water – a sure sign of excess stress, despair and anxiety – they scrabbled round the tank determined to find dry land.[206]

Grattan's team have explored the potential for prolactin to reduce anxiety in pregnant and lactating mice. During a stressful event, the hypothalamus signals to the pituitary gland via a hormone called corticotropin releasing hormone (CRH). Grattan's team found that prolactin dampened CRH neuron activity, effectively inhibiting the female's entire HPA axis.[207] This effect is thought to carry over to the weeks and months after birth when having a baby nuzzling at your breast, thus stimulating prolactin, keeps stress responses low.

Prolactin's famous cuddly cousin, oxytocin, definitely lowers stress responses when you're *not* pregnant. However, there is little evidence it does this *during* pregnancy; oxytocin's full effects don't kick in till the first labour pains. Neither oestrogen nor progesterone have a proven direct role in reducing stress during pregnancy either. Instead, a molecule called allopregnanolone, made from progesterone, ticks all the stress-reduction boxes. It's anti-stress, anti-depressive, anti-anxiety and anti-aggressive, pro-social, pro-sexual, pro-sleep and neuroprotective.

Reduced fear, stress and anxiety during pregnancy all seem like worthwhile adaptive responses. Surely a calm, chilled-out mother-to-be is preferable to a tense, worried, sleepless wreck? However, being in possession of an expectant brain, a dampened HPA axis and reduced fear response can have some unexpected emotional consequences, including increased aggression, anger and depression. This presents a conundrum: on one hand women have blunted stress responses and reduced anxiety, but at the same time we have a greater propensity for depression. This is perhaps a vital clue there is more going on in the expectant mother's mind than only 'bottom-up' hormonal signalling.

Is 'baby brain' a myth?

When this book was but a twinkle in my eye, one question gestating in my mind was: Is pregnancy truly synonymous with memory loss and ditzy docile disorganisation? Or, in other words, 'Is baby brain real?'

I'd always had my doubts.

In 2007, after five years plodding along as a postdoc, I hung up my lab coat to pursue a science writing career in a global health-communications agency. The dynamic and challenging role demanded mental sharpness, creativity and the ability to meet deadlines (academia moves at a glacial pace and when deadlines do exist, they're rarely tight). Despite being nine weeks pregnant and starving on my first day at work, I thrived, and apart from the time I nearly threw a custard pastry at a doctor, I never considered that there was a relationship between the status of my womb and my capacity to perform.

You may be expecting me to announce that 'baby brain' is yet another item on the long list of neglected themes in female brain science. Surprise! It's a very well-researched theme indeed, both in humans and non-human animals.

However, there is an intriguing paradox.

While as many as three out of every four women state they're more forgetful, 'foggy', or lack concentration during pregnancy or in the early years of motherhood,[208] the bulk of research doesn't support their experience. Most studies find pregnancy and motherhood have no effect on memory, and in plenty of studies find pregnancy *improves* cognition.

Professor Dave Grattan goes so far as saying that baby brain is one of the great myths in the field of maternal neuroscience. 'All of the evidence suggests the contrary,' he said. 'Pregnant people and animals perform better than non-mothers in all aspects of learning and memory both during pregnancy and postpartum.' As he points out, all the chemical indicators of pregnancy are all geared towards mental sharpness and good mood. Pregnant brains are flooded with the feel-good chemicals oxytocin and prolactin, and 1000-fold higher than usual levels of the cognitive enhancer oestrogen.

A 2014 study dispelling the myth of baby brain was published in *The Journal of Clinical and Experimental Neuropsychology*. Researchers were curious how memory and attention changed with pregnancy and childbirth. They recruited forty-two pregnant women, and had them complete a comprehensive battery of neuropsychological tests. Women were tested for verbal and spatial memory, attention, language skills, executive abilities and mood, and testing was repeated three and six months after babies were born.[209]

For every neuropsychological test, including memory, pregnant women and mothers performed equally as well as a matched group of 21 child-free women. There were only two significant differences between pregnancy and motherhood versus being childfree. The first was mood – as you might expect, pregnancy and motherhood lowered mood. The second was *self-reported* memory. Pregnant women and mothers consistently claimed their memory was poor or they were 'doing badly on the tests'. Surprisingly, their attitudes about poor memory persisted even when the researchers provided them with their test scores – clear evidence to the contrary. 'I was surprised at how strong the feeling was that they weren't performing well,' said Michael Larson, lead author of the study.

This type of result has been replicated numerous times. One Australian study found that despite their belief they were suffering 'baby brain', pregnant women performed better on tests of memory than non-pregnant women. 'Pregnancy may confer an advantage in memory rather than a deficit and women's complaints of memory performance may be influenced by "false expectations"', concluded the researchers.[210] Another study found that what changed with pregnancy wasn't cognitive skills but 'the women's perception of themselves'.[211]

Why do so many pregnant women say they suffer from 'baby brain' when objective testing concludes the opposite?

Katherine Ellison is a journalist who has written an entire book on the phenomenon of 'baby brain'. In *The Mommy Brain: How Motherhood Makes Us Smarter*, Ellison explains the notion arose in the 1960s when women entered the workplace in droves.[212] 'This change brought new scrutiny from others – and a new self-consciousness for mothers,' she writes. Ellison suggests that blaming 'baby brain' is our current cop-out for when we inevitably find our attention divided or we relax our guard, even for a moment. Baby brain is 'our frequent alibi when we say something dumb', and we're supported in this pessimistic belief by three out of four of our friends. The myth persists because of confirmation bias, whereby we selectively look for evidence that supports the cultural expectation. We're trained to expect to forget, so when we do we've got a ready-made reason why.

Reading the 'baby brain' literature, I'm reminded of Sarah Romans' findings concerning cultural beliefs and stereotypes around the emotional rollercoaster of hormones, menstrual cycles and PMS. It seems to me that 'baby brain' is another expectation we've absorbed without question. Larson and his team also muse over the power of cultural stereotypes in their paper and suggest the belief emphasising cognitive decline as 'inevitable' with pregnancy is related to 'the perception of a woman as emotional and at the mercy of their hormones during their menstrual cycle'.

To be fair, there are studies that find small reductions in memory or attention for some women in the third trimester of pregnancy, and especially and unsurprisingly in the first few postpartum days when the shock of childbirth is fresh and sleep is hard to come by. Sleep is key for healthy cognitive function, and we know the later stages of pregnancy are accompanied by restless nights. The combination of cortisol keeping you hyper-alert, an uncomfortable bump, aching joints softened by relaxin, and the nervous anticipation of the impending arrival is a cocktail recipe for insomnia and consequent forgetfulness.

For balance, let's consider a few alternative explanations for the paradox. Namely, the proposition that the problem isn't with women's perceptions – rather, it's with how memory is tested in the lab.

Some researchers have argued that 'baby brain' or 'brain fog' might simply be too difficult to measure in a research setting.

In the next chapter you'll learn that a similar paradox exists for sleep – though women complain they've had a terrible night's sleep, laboratory tests reveal they slept soundly. One idea is that laboratory tests aren't calibrated to pick up the nuanced changes in cognition that women are very attuned to. Perhaps inviting weary pregnant women or exhausted new mothers to sit quietly alone in a room to complete a structured recall test doesn't quite match the reality of keeping mentally sharp and on the ball in the everyday real world. They probably relish the peace and quiet, and as such ace the tests!

Pregnancy and motherhood, especially the first time around, refocus your attention inwards. Back in the 1950s, English paediatrician Donald Winnicott famously termed refocused attention 'primary maternal preoccupation … a condition of heightened sensitivity in which the mother focuses on the infant to the exclusion of all else'. In their classic book *The Birth of a Mother: How the Motherhood Experience Changes You Forever*, Daniel Stern and Nadia Bruschweiler-Stern write about the entirely new mindset of mothers: 'The motherhood mindset pushes her pre-existing mental life aside and rushes forward to fill the centre stage of her inner life, giving it a different make up entirely.'[213]

I may have a touch of confirmation bias based on my experiences, but I'm of the same mind as Ellison and Larson. 'Somebody might learn about this and say, "I am thinking okay even though I am pregnant." It might improve their quality of life, it might improve how they are functioning – they might start believing in themselves,' says Larson. Ellison states, 'Mommy Brain should be thought of less as a cerebral handicap and more as an advantage in the lifelong task of becoming smart.' Imagine if the research supported the cultural myth and was co-opted to discriminate against pregnant women and mothers in the workplace. Let's do ourselves a favour and rewrite the story.

Are labour pains needed for brain gains?

My second-born loves to hear the story of his birth. I suspect it's because Bear Grylls has a walk-on role. I'll save you all the details, but one evening while I was eating a bowl of gnocchi and green pesto watching Bear do outdoorsy upside-down things involving logs and river crossings, I felt a painful yet familiar twinge. 'Oh, yes, now I remember,' I thought to myself. 'Mum was right!' Mum had always told me when she went into labour with my younger sister the first contraction brought labour memories flooding back. For most women, the pain of labour is ranked as severe, but memories dim over time. It turns out there's nothing like those first few contractions to remind you.

I was ten days early when I went into labour the second time round, but like every pregnant woman ever, I'd already Googled 'Tips to jump start labour' and had come across all the usual ideas: curry, pineapple, acupuncture, sex, nipple squeezing, walking, and my yoga teacher taught me a 'labour induction haka' which involved a lot of deep squatting, stomping and huffing. No-one really knows what triggers labour. Medical science offers as many options as Google, and plenty of researchers are working on the issue, especially for the prevention of pre-term labour. The timing involves complex interactions between mother, baby and the placenta. What needs to happen is a shift in balance from a quiescent uterus and tightly closed cervix to a contracting uterus and soft dilated cervix and, of course, a baby mature enough to face the world.

Every woman's experience of pain during labour varies greatly. I went into my first birth assuming I'd be like my sister and the pain would be 'good pain'. I was floored when it wasn't!

Some women (like my sister) feel less pain while others find the pain extremely distressing (me).

The story goes that a 'natural' vaginal delivery sets off a cascade of hormones, which are necessary for feelings of love and tenderness towards your baby. Love is your 'reward' for labour pain. Skin-to-skin contact and breastfeeding immediately upon delivery nurture this sequence. You may have heard that the same cascade is absent when Caesarean section or pain relief is used. Or you may have heard, as I did during a conference I recently attended, that women should 'lean in to the pain of childbirth' because doing otherwise is 'denying your divine feminine' and 'rejecting your role as mother'. (The speaker was a man. And I made plenty of disparaging snorty sounds at the back of the room.)

Contemplating the relative contributions of the events surrounding birth (nature) versus interactions between mother and infant (nurture) is walking-on-eggshells territory. Typically, most studies have limitations, but the bigger problem I see is that they get co-opted and used to fuel guilt among mothers who, for whatever reason, didn't give birth 'the way nature intended'. For example, one study used fMRI to compare the brains of mothers who delivered vaginally versus via Caesarean section. During the first month postpartum, mothers from the vaginal-delivery group exhibited greater neural responses to their own babies' cries compared to mothers who delivered via Caesarean section. However, the difference between the groups of mothers disappeared by three to four months postpartum.[214]

Certainly, there is evidence that Caesarean birth delays skin-to-skin contact and breastfeeding, but only by minutes or hours. Although there may sometimes be short-term effects, the way your baby comes into the world doesn't impact on maternal feelings. It's entirely possible to feel ambivalent towards your baby after vaginal birth, or completely consumed with love after a Caesarean section.

Similarly, there is no good evidence that choosing an epidural (as I did) interferes with breastfeeding or maternal feelings (it didn't for me). There is no critical period or requirement for pain to be felt by the mother via which the mother–infant bond becomes activated.[215] Certainly, having a baby come out of your vagina doesn't flick a 'mummy switch' on in your brain.

If I think about the gorgeous group of women in my mothers' group, there's no way you'd have been able to divide us into two groups based on the quality of our parenting and birth method – vaginal-birth-loving mothers and detached Caesarean birthers (to even suggest so would be met with some serious eye rolls and sharp words).

Suffice to say, for all Mother Nature's provisions to ensure labour, delivery and maternal affection, she is neither benevolent nor benign. Today, many women are in the privileged position of being able to override her wishes with modern science-based medicine, which massively ups the ante in favour of maternal and newborn safety, survival and reduced birth trauma. And if you so choose, you can labour pain free.

Pregnancy and childbirth may provide the neural scaffold upon which maternal behaviours are built, but human parenting is not hormone *dependent*. The *experience* of nurturing a baby stimulates the hormones oxytocin and prolactin without the need for pregnancy and childbirth. This is the case for fathers, non-birth parents and other family members. It is via the act of nurturing that attachments form and love grows.

This is why babies cry

Immediately following birth, non-human animals instinctively care for their young, feed them and defend them. Typically, we do too – we smother our baby with kisses, count their fingers and toes, and soak in their delicious newborn smell. We become captivated with our babe, a process not dissimilar to falling in love.

As I've mentioned, pregnancy hormones are not necessary for successful attachment and parenting. Even virgin rats can learn how to mother simply by practising. One of the classic studies in the field showed that when standoffish virgin rats were continuously housed with strange pups, they eventually showed maternal behaviours: they retrieved pups to a single location, licked them, built nests and adopted a nursing posture over them despite not lactating. It took seven to ten days of 'pup exposure', but with experience non-birth mothers eventually learned how to care. Subsequent studies building on this finding showed that pregnancy and birth simply reduce the amount of time it takes to induce caregiving behaviours – birth mothers 'mother' immediately; fathers and non-birth mothers eventually form very close attachments too. It just takes a little patience and time.[216]

Because babies are born with an innate and powerful biological need to be loved, they behave in ways that ensure the formation of that bond. Before she can hold your gaze, smile or use her words to let you know what's wrong, crying is a baby's most powerful tool of communication. And one of the ways in which a newborn elicits a response from her parent or caregiver is by crying.

All babies cry. And from your infant's point of view, crying is essential for her survival.

Indeed, all newborn mammals cry, and different species, including humans, produce remarkably similar sounds. So much so, playing the sound of a wailing infant from one species will bring adults from another species running. One study found that wild adult deer responded to the cries of baby marmots, seals, cats, bats and humans. When I played my cocker spaniel the recording supplied by researchers he too pricked up his ears then bounded over to sniff at my laptop.[217] The theory goes that all adult mammals are 'wired to respond' to a baby crying.

Investigations typically use fMRI to test a mother's brain response to their own versus another infant's cries. Nearly every study of human parents finds that the regions that thin during pregnancy become activated when listening to infant wails. A handful of studies have found fathers respond to babies' cries too. (Who knew?) Maternal brain researcher Ruth Feldman found greater amygdala activation in mothers versus greater cortical activation in fathers in response to their infant's tears. Feldman suggests that while the hormones of pregnancy may chart a unique 'bottom-up' limbic path to mothering, in fathers paternal care is constructed in a top-down and outside-in fashion via the experience of parenting.[218]

Interacting with their children increases oxytocin, prolactin, cortisol and even oestrogen in men. Testosterone levels decline in 'hands-on' fathers, either in response to or to facilitate empathy and caregiving.[219] In terms of hormones and parenting, it's hard to tease out cause and effect. Nonetheless, interacting with babies seems to modulate their fathers' hormones and activate neural circuitry in ways that are similar to those in mothers.

This is your brain on breastfeeding

'He was born to feed,' was the first comment made by a midwife about my firstborn son, 'and so are those nipples!' I've often reminded my eldest of that comment over the years (about his ability, not mine); he's still a good eater and is famous for religiously scoffing eight or nine Weet-Bix every morning. I've tried to marinate in the praise lavished on my bosom, but I find it's not something I can easily bring up as a humble brag (although this book has finally given me a vehicle to do so).

If you've given birth, it's likely those around you will have developed a closer than usual relationship with your breasts. We're mammals, after all, and the defining feature of all female mammals is our ability to produce milk and feed it to our offspring. Of course, breastfeeding doesn't come naturally to every mother and baby, therefore a disclaimer: in the next few paragraphs I may use the term 'maternal behaviours' as an umbrella term that includes lactation. This does not imply that women who choose to bottlefeed, or who can't breastfeed, or parents who don't have breasts, or any other loving, affectionate carer of a child are not exhibiting 'maternal behaviours'. Breast may be 'best' (as the WHO states) but a happy, healthy baby is a fed baby, wherever that milk comes from.

Pregnancy prepares our brains and our breasts for motherhood. Our bosoms grow and alveoli (milk ducts) develop under the influence of oestrogen and prolactin. High oestrogen and progesterone levels prevent actual milk production, but delivery of the placenta resulting in a sudden drop in their levels results in milk 'coming in'.

After birth, breasts and alveoli continue to grow and the maintenance of milk production and the control of milk let-down remain under hormonal control. But those hormones are now under control of your baby. Suckling stimulates oxytocin that causes smooth muscle contraction and ejection of milk. In time, the mere thought of feeding your baby stimulates the extraordinary sensation of let-down. Suckling also stimulates prolactin, which maintains milk production. Importantly, oxytocin and prolactin act in the brain to modulate behaviours, thoughts and feelings.

Breastfeeding mothers differ in a few subtle ways from non-lactating parents. They report lower stress and negative moods, more sensitivity to positive emotional cues and less sensitivity to negative, threat-related cues and anxiety than non-breastfeeding mothers.[220] Lowered anxiety is matched by changes in heart-rate variability, reduced blood pressure and reduced cortisol responses to stress.

Have you heard the saying 'Never come between a mother bear and her cubs'? This is an apt description of a breastfeeding mother. In one study, researchers recruited forty mothers with babies aged three to six months, half of whom were exclusively breastfeeding. Women were assessed using measures of anger, aggression and hostility including psychological interviews and a 'set-up' where a researcher posing as another mother provoked hostile reactions during a game. Mothers who exclusively breast-fed their infants were almost *twice* as aggressive as women who weren't breastfeeding. They also had lower blood pressure, which was taken as an indication of lowered arousal and reduced stress response.[221]

When a mother bear lashes out at an intruder, her response is called 'lactation aggression' or 'maternal defence'. While it might sound counterintuitive, aggression is an 'approach behaviour'. If your baseline stress and fear levels are low, you're braver and more able to get up close and in someone's face.

I clearly recall my first 'mother bear' response about two days after my first son was born and a nurse came to perform his heel prick, a harmless blood test that screens for a variety of genetic disorders. Predictably, he screamed and my response to his pain was instantaneous and primal. I had to hold myself back from shoving the nurse away and curling myself over his little body to keep him safe. After she left all I could do was cry, partly in empathy at his pain but mostly because it had dawned on me that I was a mother, and I was behaving in ways I didn't recognise.

Breastfeeding and the neural control of fertility

Around the same day as the heel-prick incident, I dutifully went along to a postnatal education class run by the hospital midwives. I was sitting very gingerly on one bum cheek when, much to the bemusement of the room, the topic of postpartum contraception was raised (by a midwife, not a fresh new mum). In addition to the usual methods of contraception (the pill, IUDs, condoms and the like) we were told about the lactational amenorrhoea method (LAM). LAM is a natural birth control technique based on the fact that lactation causes amenorrhoea (lack of menstruation). It's Mother Nature's way of providing a natural delay in your return to fertility and spacing babies more optimally.

Here's the theory of why, in a perfect scenario, LAM works: a suckling baby stimulates the release of prolactin. Prolactin blocks kisspeptin and GnRH (*tick-tick-tick*), thus suppressing ovulation. No ovulation means no chance of an egg-meets-sperm (locks in and is the winner!) event.

Some non-pregnant or non-breastfeeding people (males and females) make too much prolactin, known medically as hyperprolactinaemia. If you produce too much prolactin you're rendered infertile. One common cause is a type of pituitary tumour that secretes excessive levels of prolactin; other times the cause is genetic. In women hyperprolactinaemia prevents ovulation and menstruation, and causes infertility and sometimes milk production without pregnancy. Some infertility drugs bypass prolactin and kisspeptin to stimulate GnRH release directly, and some researchers are exploring the potential for kisspeptin as an infertility treatment.[222]

The WHO that states breastfeeding is ninety-eight per cent effective in preventing pregnancy, but only if you're able to answer 'yes' to these three questions:

1. Have you had a period since your baby was born?
2. Is your baby less than six months old?
3. Are you nursing your baby on demand day and night, and waiting no longer than four hours between feedings during the day and six hours between feedings at night, with no pacifiers or supplementary bottles?

Fail to answer 'Yes' to all three and you'll need an alternative method of contraception (unless you're planning another pregnancy). Some proponents such as La Leche League claim that mothers who closely follow the LAM 'tenets of ecological breastfeeding' will experience an average of fourteen months menstruation free. Of course, these criteria may or may not be achievable for every family, so LAM is not recommended as a fail-safe method. Mother Nature is not infallible.

Depression and motherhood

Pregnancy and motherhood made me feel like I'd finally joined the human race. But at the same time, I didn't have a clue who I was anymore. I've often commented that it wasn't looking after my boys that made motherhood so emotionally challenging, it was managing myself. Motherhood is viewed as both a natural and sacred role – the epitome of bliss, serenity and fulfilment as a woman. For many women it is nothing of the sort.

In chapter 6, I described some reasons for the gender gap in anxiety and depression. Skewing the stats are the uniquely female experiences of pregnancy and motherhood. Your emotions ensure you're sensitive to your baby's needs, but brain plasticity comes at a cost and leaves you vulnerable to developing mood disorders.

The baby blues

In my postnatal education classes, the focus was very much on the days and weeks immediately following birth as the vulnerable window for mood disorders. There is voluminous information on antenatal and postpartum depression, including plenty of cookie-cutter advice on mental health prevention – ask for help, sleep when baby sleeps, eat well and exercise.

We hear a lot about postnatal depression (PND), but far less about depression *during* pregnancy. Antenatal depression, as it's called, affects around one in ten mothers during their pregnancy. Reasons for feeling blue, deeply depressed or anxious during pregnancy vary, but are not dissimilar to the causes at other times of life: combinations of lack of social support and a good dose of rumination, stressful life events, the thought of impending motherhood, but with the addition of hormonal change. Women who've suffered mood disorders before falling pregnant are the most vulnerable to antenatal depression.[223]

First-week baby blues are most likely due to the dramatic withdrawal from the high levels of hormones produced by the placenta. There's a sort of postpartum swing away from feel-good neurotransmitters and hormones, and a swing towards those that induce low mood. In principle, oxytocin and prolactin as a result of breastfeeding and loving your newborn should buffer low postnatal mood (all good in theory, clearly not always good in practice!).

The thing is, motherhood doesn't magically become carefree and joyous after baby's first birthday. If anything, the years that follow continue to wear you down bit by bit, making the emergence of mood disorders more likely than in the early postpartum months.

This concept has support from the Australian Longitudinal Study on Women's Health (ALSWH) which, since the 1990s, has followed 58 000 women born in the 1920s, 1950s and 1970s. A survey of 9145 women in the 1970s cohort found that mothers with older children (over twelve months) reported lower scores of wellbeing and mental health than women with babies under twelve months.[224] That is, the longer women were mothers, the worse their mental health.

Depression and the myths of motherhood

How can motherhood – sold to us as a woman's most fulfilling and rewarding life experience – be connected to the development of depression?

Daniel Stern argues that the birth of a mother does not take place in one dramatic defining moment but 'gradually emerges from the cumulative work of the many months that precede and follow the actual birth of the baby'. In a sense, a mother is 'born psychologically much as her baby is born physically', he writes. 'What a woman gives birth to in her mind is not a new human being but a new identity and sense of being a mother.'[213]

Children bring about a change in your priorities, your relationships and the identity you've very carefully constructed since girlhood. The transformation to motherhood is often filled with deep dissatisfaction, resentment, guilt, shame and even ambivalence. I certainly found myself conflicted by my expectations and my experiences of motherhood.

To explore the conflict between the myths and realities, Professor Jane Ussher conducted a series of interviews with women, concentrating on mothers whose eldest child was aged between one and three. She was curious if motherhood was what they expected it to be. She interviewed women with older children because she hoped they'd no longer be caught up with the minutiae of baby care, and they might reflect more clearly on the practical and psychological changes of motherhood. Also, these women should still have reasonably clear memories of life before kids.[225]

For all women, the reality of motherhood was 'totally different' from what they had expected. Women became disillusioned on two counts, she says: by discovering that motherhood had overwhelmed, rather than enhanced, their identities as women, and by 'finding that the dominant societal discourses of motherhood were misleading'. The sheer drudgery of parenting exposed the popular images of the 'attractive, perfectly dressed and made-up mother, with her happy, smiling family' as a myth. 'Motherhood did not equate with womanhood, as expected, it engulfed it,' writes Ussher.

Ussher and others have proposed that it's the disillusionment arising from the conflict between the myth and reality that causes depression, especially if there are other problems and pressures.

Motherhood for me has been a case study in resolving the conflict between myth and reality. I only wish I'd learned sooner that my experience wasn't quite so unique.

Once a mother, always a mother

Motherhood is the one relationship guaranteed to irrevocably alter us. As we build lives for 'we' not 'me', we learn that life's ups and downs, milestones, opportunities and risks are enmeshed with other people. Parenting requires us to repeatedly deploy cognitive skills such as planning, organisation, working memory, flexibility, attention and decision-making. We practise and refine empathy, emotional regulation and resilience. All the evidence from non-human animals suggests that motherhood bestows a cognitive advantage. Mothers also live longer and are protected against brain ageing. As we'll discuss in the final chapter of this book, there is evidence for a link between motherhood, good health and longevity.

Sheila Kitzinger, the famous childbirth educator and social anthropologist, writes, 'Childbirth might be the grand finale of pregnancy, but it opens the door on a completely new experience, and lengthy learning process that never finishes however old the children are.' She has a point. Parenting is a process (I'm tempted to use the word 'journey'), and at each stage of our children's development we're faced with new challenges, decisions to make, dilemmas to solve and new emotional storms to navigate. Rather like a brain-training game, parenting pushes us to upskill with each new level.

9.

Menopause

APOLOGIES. I REALISE WE'VE SKIPPED FROM MOTHERHOOD TO menopause; from fecundity to the free-fall of fertility, without a break in which to enjoy midlife. (For what it's worth, I considered inserting the chapter on mental health here, but that seemed a rather depressing option.) As I write this chapter, I too find myself rather reluctantly in the early stages of 'midlife', what I've come to think of as the old age of youth and the youth of old age. My oldest son has been earth-side for a decade, but menopause still seems like something my mother once did with her friends, certainly not something that will become a reality for me within the next few years.

Older friends have told me that menopause is the last taboo, and there certainly seems to be a stigma talking about the 'climacteric' (as it's sometimes called). Rather like 'period dramas', most of the menopausal stories are extraordinarily negative. I've heard stories of take-the-world-in-their-stride women giving up work, previously upbeat women being prescribed antidepressants, divorce, lost libidos, fear of 'cancer-causing' hormone therapies, and duelling hormonal houses where pubertal teens and menopausal mothers collide. One friend told me about the incredible panic attacks she's started experiencing. British artist Tracey Emin commented, 'It's horrible … it is the beginning of dying,' and Oprah spoke of her life force 'being slowly drained'.

Burying my head in the literature, I've found that, as with puberty, periods and labour pain, when it comes to menopause we're all different. As Kaz Cooke writes, one woman's 'power-surging goddess-affirming blessed-relief graduation from her reproductive years' is another woman's 'nasty hormonal nightmare hot-flashy forgetting faff-about, complete with mad spotty periods'.[226] My balm has been my mum who, despite being famous in our family for her sensitivity to hot and cold, didn't find the experience as troubling as some of her friends (thankfully, women and their daughters and sisters often have similar timing and experiences of menopause).

I've learned that about twenty per cent of women will have symptoms so severe that they significantly interfere with daily life; another twenty per cent will sail through with no symptoms at all, leaving sixty per cent of women experiencing mild to moderate symptoms. Your genes, general level of health and wellbeing, previous experience of mood problems, cultural expectations, exposure to stressful life events, and whether your menopause is natural, surgical or chemotherapy-induced all impact the experience.

The good news is that once you move from peri-menopause (the years leading up to your last period) into post-menopause, hormones level out and symptoms typically settle. The Melbourne Women's Midlife Health Project has found that most women report a *greater* sense of wellbeing, better moods, less depression and even a better sex life in their fifties and sixties. For many women, late midlife means children have left the nest and they discover a renewed lust for life and the confidence to be themselves regardless of the opinions or reactions of others.[227]

Whether you experience a gentle goddess path or horrible hormonal hell, menopause signifies the end of fertility. As your ovaries wind down their duties and head towards retirement, the ovarian-brain conversation falters, then disconnects altogether. We tend to think of menopause as the final reproductive life transition, but the symptoms of hot flashes, changes in sleep, mood and memory are largely due to changes in the brain. Menopause opens a window of neural vulnerability for the development of mood disorders, insomnia and cognitive change. It's when bottom-up biology (running out of eggs) paves the way for outside-in and top-down risk factors to wield a little more power than normal.

There are hundreds of books, articles and online resources on the menopausal transition. Rather than repeating much of that information, in this chapter I'll describe 'the change' from a brain health perspective with a particular focus on the neurobiology of hot flashes, sleep, mood and memory. In the second half of this chapter, I'll explore various treatments with a focus on hormone therapies (including hormone replacement therapy – HRT) for symptoms of menopause. I'll take a look at the historical controversies and the current best practice evidence-based advice being given to women.

A quick guide to the stages of menopause

In Australia, the average age for natural menopause is fifty-one, but it can occur earlier or later. If you have your last period before the age of forty you've experienced 'premature menopause', although sometimes this is referred to as 'primary ovarian insufficiency'. 'Early menopause' is when your last period happens before the age of forty-five. Menopause may also happen as a result of chemotherapy or radiotherapy treatment for cancer, or when ovaries are removed surgically (oophorectomy). In the case of surgical menopause, hormone levels drop rapidly, and severe menopause symptoms may be triggered within days.

Menopause is defined as twelve consecutive months without a menstrual period. Every day that follows is post-menopause, a phase that can make up a third of your life or more. Perimenopause ('around menopause') is defined as the years leading up to menopause, and it can start five to ten years before your last period. Menopause happens because you eventually run out of eggs, and the wide age range during which women reach menopause (anywhere between forty to fifty-eight years – fifty-one is just the average) reflects numbers of eggs and the rate of egg loss, which varies greatly between women.[228]

Perimenopause is physiologically different from post-menopause. During perimenopause, the HPO axis that has been running smoothly since menarche starts to sputter and, as such, the time is characterised by erratic and unpredictable hormone production. Gynaecologist Tara Allmen says in her excellent book *Menopause Confidential* that during perimenopause our ovaries can still make oestrogen, but just not reliably and in the right quantity. 'Sometimes they make too much oestrogen. Sometimes they make too little. And other times they get it just right.' There is no month-to-month predictability as to how oestrogen production will perform. It's the rollercoaster of ovarian hormones in perimenopause, rather than the flat tramline of post-menopause, that causes many of the 'menopausal' symptoms.

You could liken menopause to puberty in reverse. Unlike puberty, the brain is not the conductor of the menopausal orchestra. Instead, dwindling egg supplies direct the final performance. In time, the brain – like the body – learns to function without oestrogen. Women living well decades past their menopause are testament to this fact.

Why do we go through menopause?

Our rodent friends, who do so much sacrificial work to inform us about our own brains, also undergo a reproductive senescence. Ageing female rats show a decline in egg numbers, irregular cycling, irregular fertility, hormone fluctuations and insensitivity to oestrogen. Then they die. As do almost all female mammals once they're no longer fertile.

Healthy human women can expect to live a good thirty to forty years following reproductive senescence. Besides humans, we know of only two other species of mammals that live well past their reproductive prime: orca whales (also known as killer whales) and short-finned pilot whales.

Why do women (and some whales) go through menopause but not die?

The most popular idea is the 'grandmother theory', which proposes that the wise grandma contributes to her 'genetic legacy' by living on to help her grandchildren survive and thrive by sharing wisdom. Grandmothers babysit and remember tribal lore about how to live through floods, famines and other hardships. If grandmothers remained fertile, they'd be busy selfishly raising infants of their own and would be less likely to devote time to the tribe.

It's been suggested that menopause in humans is simply an artefact of our modern lifestyles – we live longer thanks to modern medicine. But a famous 2015 study published in *Current Biology* supports the 'grandmother as wise matriarch' notion.[229] The authors reported on a nine-year study of orcas that spend their summers wallowing in the waters off the southern tip of Vancouver Island in Canada. Like humans, orcas breed between the ages of twelve and forty, go through menopause, then survive well into their nineties. Using the knowledge and experience built up over many summers, the wise menopausal matriarchs took on important leadership roles in their pod. They were the ones in charge of leading others to find salmon, particularly when the fish were scarce, and their pods thrived. In short: mothers breed, grandmothers feed.

Are your menopause symptoms all in your head?

Many women transition through menopause without any health issues and remain healthy in the decades that follow. Some women, however, become vulnerable to the neurological shifts that can occur during the transition and are thus at increased risk of unhealthy brain ageing.

If you've experienced menopause, it may come as no surprise to you that oestrogen receptors (which are now looking a little empty and neglected) are found in the same brain regions that regulate temperature, sex drive, sleep, emotions, attention and memory. Changes in oestrogen signalling (either through changes in oestrogen levels or changes in oestrogen receptors) will directly affect how these numerous brain circuits function, although the exact mechanisms by which menopause alters brain physiology to generate symptoms isn't clear.

One working hypothesis focuses on the metabolic link between oestrogen and healthy cell function. Our brains metabolise twenty per cent of our energy supplies, and the brain's main fuel supply is glucose. In women, oestrogen supports the biochemical pathways that use insulin and generate energy from glucose. So the menopausal drop in oestrogen might change how efficiently the brain uses glucose and in turn how well neurons function.[230]

The link between oestrogen and glucose metabolism plays out more clearly in women who have their ovaries removed before they go through menopause – the abrupt drop in oestrogen levels is associated with an increased risk of developing Type 2 diabetes. The same increased risk for Type 2 diabetes is seen after natural menopause, whereas for women using hormone therapy, glucose metabolism is typically normal.[230, 231] I'll save the lifestyle lecture for another time, but the link between oestrogen, glucose metabolism and Type 2 diabetes highlights the importance of self-care and attention to exercise and healthy eating for women as they age.

This is your brain on hot flashes

Hot flashes (also called hot flushes) are the most common menopausal symptom and some say the defining feature of the fertility free-fall. Roughly seventy-five to eighty per cent of women experience what doctors call 'vasomotor symptoms'. For some, they're the one and only symptom. For others, they occur alongside insomnia, depression and brain fog.

Hot flashes may feel like a full-body experience but they're regulated by that busiest of brain regions, the hypothalamus. Body temperature is regulated between set thresholds within a few tenths of a degree above or below 37°C by warm-sensitive neurons in the pre-optic area of the hypothalamus, which increase or decrease their firing rate in response to rises or falls in core temperature. We have an upper threshold for heat and a lower threshold for cold. Much like a neural thermostat, the hypothalamus detects when our core temperature crosses one of these thresholds and signals the body into action. If you're too hot you'll sweat, your blood vessels will vasodilate and you'll flush red (my personal speciality), you'll want to take off a few layers of clothes, or kick off the bedsheets. And if you're too cold you'll shiver, seek warmth and/or go looking for a spare jumper.

During menopause, your upper 'hot' threshold level moves down and the lower 'cool' threshold moves up, so your thermostat narrows and becomes rather more sensitive to even tiny variations in core temperature. You'll sweat *and* shiver more easily.

The importance of ovarian hormones in what scientists call 'thermoregulation' went unrecognised for decades because researchers were far too busy studying fit, sweating men. Except for one study in 1940 by physiologist James Hardy, women were typically excluded from thermoregulation research.[232] Hardy believed men had a narrower threshold for sweating and shivering than women because in the cold women's extra body fat kept them warm, and 'in the warm zone long before women have started to perspire or even "glow", the men may be covered in beads of sweat'. For many years thereafter it was wrongly assumed women had a wider comfort zone because of our biology. We also had a lower capacity for exercise (it strained our delicate hearts, a reason also given for banning women from competing in marathons), and for excitement (men were the sweaty explorers of jungles and deserts while women stayed home, coolly and calmly minding children).

Our current understanding of thermoregulation indicates that sex differences are actually quite tiny when physical fitness and body size are taken into account. Fit and excitable women have very well-functioning thermoregulatory systems that enable us to cool down when necessary, thank you very much.[233]

This is an important point: the fitter you are, the more efficient your thermoregulation system. Exercise doesn't reduce the number of hot flashes, but being fit and healthy does make them much more bearable.

Hormones warm us up and cool us down

If you've ever taken your temperature daily to monitor your fertility and estimate ovulation timing, you'll be familiar with how your basal body temperature shifts across your cycle. Prior to ovulation, oestrogen keeps your body temperature low by promoting sweating, flushing and loss of body heat. Progesterone, which is manufactured by the corpus luteum after ovulation, reduces sweating and flushing, so you retain heat and warm up.

Oestrogen tweaks the thermostat settings, which is why treating women with oestrogen reduces hot flashes.[231] Exactly how diminishing ovarian hormone levels narrow the hypothalamic thermostat is a mystery (yes, another gap in our neuro-knowledge). We have receptors for oestrogen throughout our bodies, so changing levels of oestrogens and progesterone may also directly influence the control of skin blood flow. But, once again, very little is known about such mechanisms.[233]

One theory involves kisspeptin. Recall in chapter 3, I discussed how puberty begins with a 'kiss' when KNDy neurons in the hypothalamus switch on. The same neurons form synapses with warm-sensitive neurons in the hypothalamus. During menopause, KNDy neurons swell up, which changes the way warm-sensitive neurons respond to temperature. Lending support to this idea, a new drug treatment for hot flashes that works by blocking the KNDy–kisspeptin pathway has recently been successfully trialled.[234]

Given their regularity and reliability, hot flashes are easily studied using fMRI. Women lie on a heating pad in the scanner and are gently toasted until a hot flash is inevitably triggered. Rather surprisingly, the hypothalamus is not always active during a hot flash. This could be due to resolution issues – it may not be possible to image the quick-fire activity of only a few thousand neurons based on large-scale changes in blood flow. Alternatively, all our theories based on human hypothalamic thermostats may be wrong![235]

The brain isn't silent during hot flashes, and in many women the insular and anterior cingulate cortices activate as they feel their 'power surge'. The insular cortex perceives feelings and sensations from our bodies that relate to wellbeing, energy, mood and temperament. It processes how we *feel* about what we're feeling. Seems rather fitting, wouldn't you say?

This is your brain on disrupted sleep

When I asked the women in my book club what they struggled with most during their change of life, almost all responded with one word: sleep. I love to sleep. I power nap daily, and usually head off to bed around 9 p.m. with a good book. Not a lot gets between my pillow and me (just ask my husband), so the prospect of disrupted sleep makes me very nervous about the decade ahead.

A search of the literature supports the experiences of my book club: forty to sixty per cent of menopausal women report problems with sleep, the most common complaint being waking up at night for no apparent reason.[236] One in three perimenopausal women say sleep problems caused them distress and impacts their daytime functioning, which pretty much qualifies them for a diagnosis of insomnia.[237]

Curiously, in women but not men sleep is partially regulated by sex hormones. So it should come as no surprise sleep disruptions strike during times of hormonal transition such as puberty, pregnancy and menopause, and during the menstrual cycle. One-third of women complain of sleep disturbances and related symptoms during their periods because of cramps, heavy bleeding, bloating and headaches.

Problems with sleep may cause brain fog (more on that shortly), be caused by hot flashes, and be both the cause and consequence of mood disorders.

A quick guide to the neurobiology of sleep

Like all creatures, we evolved internal biological clocks that are synchronised by the rising and setting of the sun and determine daily rhythms including our sleep–wake cycles. Our modern technology-driven lives have us ritually underconsuming natural light during the day, overconsuming artificial light at night, and devaluing the fundamental importance of sleep. We tend to forget that we too are earthlings who need to respect sunrise and sunset.

No aspect of our biology is safe from sleep deprivation. Skip one night's sleep and you feel utterly dreadful. Suffer from insomnia, regularly get insufficient sleep, or work the night shift and you're at risk of depression, metabolic disorders such as Type 2 diabetes, cardiovascular disease, cognitive decline and a host of other health problems including increased mortality.[238]

Sleep is under the control of multiple brain systems. Our master circadian clock is located in the suprachiasmatic nucleus (SCN) of the hypothalamus. The SCN receives input from the retina, which sends signals about light and dark from the eyes. Like every cell in the body, SCN neurons also contain a twenty-four-hour clock that keeps them on track even in the absence of light or other environmental cues. The SCN is rich with receptors for oestrogen and forms circuits with other brain regions involved in arousal and attention. Other hormones, including melatonin, cortisol, thyroid-stimulating hormone and prolactin vary across the day and night, and are regulated by our circadian rhythms and sleep–wake cycles.

When we're asleep we pass through a number of sleep stages. We typically cycle from stage one (relaxation) through to four (deep restorative sleep) and back again to REM (rapid eye movement/dreaming) sleep. One 'sleep cycle' takes about ninety minutes. Typically, we have longer periods of deep sleep early in the night, and more periods of REM later in the night. Sleep studies use the tools of polysomnography to monitor sleep phases via brain waves (electroencephalography – EEG), heart rate, breathing, eye movement and leg movement. EEG electrodes attach to the scalp, and characteristic EEG patterns are associated with each stage. For example, stages three and four are marked by 'slow wave' or 'delta wave' EEG, whereas REM is characterised by 'desynchronous' or saw-tooth EEG patterns.

Sex differences in sleep

Compared to men, women are twice as likely to have trouble with sleep.[239] Before puberty, girls and boys experience problems such as trouble falling asleep at similar rates. During puberty, the prevalence of insomnia symptoms increases from 3.4 per cent to 12.2 per cent in girls (3.6-fold) and from 4.3 per cent to 9.1 per cent in boys (2.1-fold). During midlife the sleep issues and insomnia rates in women increase dramatically. Doctors remark that they're one of the most common complaints they hear about.[240]

Healthy women and men have different experiences of sleep quality.

For example, women fall asleep faster, spend more time in deep sleep, and are less likely to wake up in the middle of the night. Women's 'sleep efficiency' – the percentage of time lying down that is actually spent asleep – is greater than men's.

However, an intriguing paradox exists.

Despite women objectively experiencing better quality sleep than men, women consistently report *poorer* quality sleep. Women are more likely than men to say they have trouble falling asleep, wake at night, or upon waking feel unrested. There is a disconnect between *subjective perceptions* and *objective measures* of sleep in women.[241]

Hoping to find a more scientifically valid explanation than 'women complain more than men', I called Jessica Mong, a neuroendocrinologist and professor of pharmacology at the University of Maryland. Mong is a protégée of Margaret McCarthy, and during her postdoctoral research she made a novel observation linking oestrogen to a gene that controls sleep.

Mong believes that one reason for the apparent friction between women's reported and recorded sleep experiences lies in the small sex differences in circadian rhythms. She thinks that for some women there might be a conflict between their 'biological bedtime' and their actual bedtime.

This can best be explained by looking at the results of a 2002 study of 2135 Spanish and Italian students aged eighteen to thirty. All students filled in the 'morningness–eveningness questionnaire' (MEQ) to establish if they were an early bird, a night owl or somewhere in between. Subjects answered questions such as, 'If you got into bed at 11.00 p.m., how tired would you be?' or 'Assume that you work a five-hour day (including breaks), your job is interesting, and you are paid based on your performance. At what time would you choose to begin?' Average MEQ scores differed significantly between men and women. Women felt the need for sleep earlier in the evening than men and woke up earlier. Men preferred to go to bed later and wake later. Women reported having an earlier peak time for mental performance and time of day for 'feeling best'. (There was, however, a small d-value of 0.28 and a large degree of overlap of eighty-nine per cent.)[242]

As Mong and I discussed, this suggests some (not all) women (and some men) may head off to bed later than their 'natural bedtime' requires and despite getting a 'good night's sleep', are operating in a state of mild jetlag.

Mong suggests mood disorders also contribute to the perception of poorer sleep quality – our assessment of how well we've slept is strongly impacted by anxiety and depression. But mood doesn't fully explain the differences between perception and objective measures that exist for healthy women and men.

Another reason Mong gave for the conundrum is similar to that discussed for thermoregulation – the majority of sleep research has been done on men, and there are significant gaps in our knowledge of how biological sex influences our circadian rhythms and sleep. Because traditional laboratory recordings of sleep quality such as EEG are based on male physiology, they may not be 'tuned' to detect sleep quality in women.

Certainly the discordance between how women say they feel versus what sleep study data displays has led to a lack of clarity about the true nature of sleep and insomnia in midlife women, especially during menopause.[243]

How do ovarian hormones influence our experience of sleep? Given women's experiences of sleep at reproductive life transitions such as puberty, pregnancy and menopause, our current understanding of the relationships between circadian rhythms, sex hormones and the sleep–wake cycle in women is pretty poor. Yet another field of neuroscience in its infancy!

Which comes first – hormones, hot flashes or sleep problems?

For women going through the change of life, it would seem likely that a domino effect of sorts is the cause: hormones cause hot flashes and hot flashes cause poor sleep. However, not every woman wakes up during a night-time flash, and there is some evidence that waking up *triggers* the flashing and sweating.[243, 244] Furthermore, while HRT is the most effective treatment for those women suffering hot flashes or night sweats, not all women find that HRT helps insomnia.

There are plenty of reasons for developing sleep problems at any point in the lifespan. A combination of stress, poor lifestyle choices, medical conditions, or plain old bad habits such as taking your iPhone to bed to check Facebook impact healthy sleep.

Midlife also brings with it difficulties with work, teenage children (perhaps even a child going through puberty), potential problems with long-term relationships and ageing parents. We know poor sleep affects mood the next day, and in turn feeling anxious in turn adversely affects sleep.

A psychiatrist friend of mine says she often counsels her patients that waking up, especially as you get older, is perfectly normal. Lying there worrying that you're not getting your required unbroken eight hours (among other concerns) makes things worse. It's easy to get caught in a vicious cycle of wakefulness and worrying, with night sweats and mood disorders giving ample time for minds to ruminate in the wee hours.

Sleep problems often need to be dealt with using an armoury of therapeutic and lifestyle tools. We'll discuss the role for hormone therapy later in the chapter. Lifestyle recommendations include the usual healthy diet and physical exercise recommendations, with particular attention to 'sleep hygiene' including avoiding stimulants, keeping your bedroom dark and cool, and limiting artificial light sources after sundown.

This is your brain on the menopausal blues

For all women, but especially those with a history of clinical mood disorders, the years around the menopause are now recognised as a window of vulnerability for depression. Similar windows open at other times of intense hormonal instability or dramatic shifts in hormone levels such as puberty and postpartum.

Feeling sad, anxious, irritable or suffering mood swings are common symptoms affecting up to one in five women in midlife. Depression or anxiety is not necessarily going to develop unless you have a long-standing history of mood disorders or PMDD. If they do emerge, symptoms are much the same as those discussed previously and include emotional flatness, feeling unable to cope, irritability, social isolation, tearfulness, decreased energy and failure to enjoy normal activities and relationships.

In chapter 6 we discussed the multitude of bottom-up/biological, outside-in/social and top-down/psychological factors that influence the development of depression and anxiety. From a bottom-up perspective, it's thought that oestradiol modulates the synthesis, availability and metabolism of serotonin, a key neurotransmitter in depression, and dopamine, involved in motivation and pleasure. So menopause itself doesn't *cause* depression but the transition is when bottom-up hormones appear to be in the driving seat (or, at the very least, a loud and obnoxious back-seat driver).

Because symptoms may be gradual in onset, or fluctuate over the course of a decade or more, some women will not recognise symptoms as part of a reversible and treatable problem, but rather will interpret them as a permanent change in their life. Jayashri Kulkarni says that perimenopausal mood disorders are not well recognised and are wrongly treated with antidepressants. 'Women with this type of depression generally respond better to hormone treatments. But the link between depression and hormones is not often made,' she says. Kulkarni believes there is a great deal of variation between women in how their hormones affect mood. 'Some women are very sensitive to small shifts in gonadal hormones; others are not,' she says.[245] The good news is menopausal mood swings are not the 'new normal', they are treatable, and the blues often lift once women shift from perimenopause into late post-menopause.[246]

This is your brain on 'brain fog'

I've heard clinicians say 'brain fog' isn't a real diagnosis, which is correct. 'Brain fog' is a colloquial description of symptoms used to describe slow or hazy thinking, difficulty focusing, confusion, lack of concentration and forgetfulness. Unless someone is medically or scientifically trained, they're not going to describe their symptoms as 'similar to mild cognitive impairment' (which is the medical description).

Regardless of terminology, the menopausal transition is a time of increased vulnerability to foggy thoughts and memory issues. A meta-analysis published in 2014 confirmed that these symptoms are not imaginary. Compared to young, healthy, fertile women, post-menopausal women performed worse on tasks of verbal memory and fluency.[247] Similarly, women who'd had their ovaries surgically removed and were plunged into sudden menopause also performed worse on verbal memory tests after surgery.

Professor John Eden, gynaecologist and reproductive endocrinologist and director of the Women's Health and Research Institute of Australia, told me that a change in 'word-finding' ability is a common symptom in the menopausal women he treats. He commented that lawyers, in particular, notice this symptom early, presumably because they rely so heavily on verbal gymnastics and sharp recall.

Memory lapses and inability to concentrate may be attributed to poor-quality sleep and tiredness which become compounded by stress, mood disorders and the life circumstances women often find themselves experiencing in their late forties and fifties. Coping with teenagers, ageing parents with health problems, work, and relationship issues can all negatively impact cognitive function. Is there evidence linking 'brain fog' to dwindling ovarian hormones?

Neurally speaking, oestrogen enables sharp thinking by keeping synapses healthy. If you were to view young healthy neurons under a high-powered microscope, you'd see their dendrites are covered in tiny nubs or spines, like buds on a tree branch. As we age we lose spines. Think of a young tree in late spring growing new branches, twigs and lush foliage versus the bare branches of a tree in winter. We see loss of spines in menopausal monkeys and rodents who've had their ovaries removed, and spine loss is correlated with worse memory. We have no idea if this is also the case in menopausal women, but it's certainly a possibility that hormone decline is responsible for brain fog because of spine loss.

When writing this chapter, I had conversations with clinicians about the menopausal chicken-and-egg scenario. At best they conclude that symptoms are interlinked. 'Hot flashes and sweats, sleep disturbance, low mood and anxiety, all can have a negative impact on higher brain function,' said Sonia Davison, endocrinologist at Jean Hailes for Women's Health via email. 'You can't dissect out hot flashes and sweats from sleep disturbance. We know sleep is really important for consolidation of memory. But is brain fog due to disturbed sleep, anxiety, or hormones? We just don't know,' Professor Sue Davis from Monash University told me over the phone.

Is it 'brain fog' or dementia?

One of the fears many women have is whether their foggy brain is an early sign of an inevitable decline towards dementia. One neuroscientist I know, a dementia researcher in her late forties, confessed to me even she'd visited her GP to talk through her symptoms for fear she had early onset Alzheimer's disease (AD).

Her fears were not unfounded. Menopausal brain fog and early stage AD share many of the same symptoms, including those of which my friend had a detailed professional understanding. AD often begins with lapses in memory and difficulty in finding the right words for everyday objects.[248]

We'll unpack the various types of memory loss as a part of normal ageing, mild cognitive decline and dementia in the next chapter. For now it's important to realise that a certain degree of forgetfulness is normal at any stage of life. We all have 'tip-my-the-tongue' moments, call our children by the wrong name, or can't remember why we walked into a room. We just tend to become more conscious of 'senior moments' the older we get.

So how do you differentiate between the symptoms of cognitive decline and menopause?

'Clinically, you can't,' answered John Eden when I posed this question to him. 'The simplest way to find out is to give women two months of hormone therapy and see if their symptoms improve.'

What role does hormone therapy play in the improvement of brain fog? Similar to our foggy understanding of the role of hormones and memory loss, researchers are struggling to come up with a clear answer.

As a rule, normal memory loss involves forgetting where you put your keys, whereas dementia involves forgetting what your keys are for.

Will you 'suffer' or 'sail' through menopause?

Elsewhere in this book, I've introduced you to people who appear to be 'immune' or resilient to whatever troubles life throws their way. Children who display exceptional resilience have been likened to dandelions who grow and thrive in a crack in the concrete, in contrast to the more delicate orchids who need more careful attention to blossom. In chapter 6 we met the Dunedin Study 'seventeen per cent' who remain mentally well into midlife. And in the final chapter of this book you'll meet an exceptional group of individuals (three out of every four of whom are women) who reach the age of a hundred and beyond.

While many women 'suffer' through menopause, I was curious about the twenty per cent of women who sail through the change without encountering stormy waters. What are the traits of these women? Can doctors predict in advance who these symptom-free women will be? And what can we learn from them?

Sadly, I was unable to find any literature focusing on what I'd like to call 'menopausal dandelions'; instead, most evidence identifies risk factors for developing various menopausal symptoms (with the best characterised being insomnia and depression).

Risk factors for developing insomnia or depression during menopause include:

- ♀ Low socioeconomic status.
- ♀ Being in a minority or marginalised social group.
- ♀ Poor overall physical health.
- ♀ Experiencing psychosocial stressors.
- ♀ Personality traits of higher neuroticism, lower agreeableness, lower conscientiousness.
- ♀ A history of depression or PMDD.

Jean Hailes for Women's Health notes that how you react to menopause will depend on factors including:

- ♀ The type of menopause you have – whether it is 'natural', expected and on time, early, or as a result of surgery or chemotherapy.
- ♀ Your age.
- ♀ Your stage of life and whether you have done the things you wanted to, like have children or all the children you wanted to have.
- ♀ Whether you have achieved the things you wanted to achieve – do you have an identity and purpose you are happy with?
- ♀ How you view your body and feel about the changes that are happening to you.
- ♀ Are you as healthy as you can be and taking care of yourself?[249]

Interestingly, there is evidence for cultural differences in the experience of menopause, with different sets of symptoms reported in different countries (rather like PMS). Indigenous

Australian women may view menopause more positively, not so much as the end of their reproductive life but the beginning of their role as cultural leaders. Women from some Western cultures are more likely to view menopause negatively – it's the end of their reproductive years as well as their sexual desirability and they experience a sense of grief and loss.[249]

Hormone therapy for menopause

Hormone replacement therapy (HRT), sometimes called hormone therapy (HT), is a drug combination of oestrogen and/or progesterone, and sometimes testosterone.

Replacing hormones using HRT is the most effective treatment available for symptoms related to oestrogen withdrawal during menopause, if started when symptoms begin, that is, before the age of sixty or within ten years of menopause.[250, 251]

For many women, the decision to use HRT remains a scary one. While writing this chapter, most women I spoke to were terrified of the risks and unsure about the benefits.

The choice to use any type of HRT, including the contraceptive pill, is not simple because there are complicated risks and benefits to weigh up, confusing messages and newspaper reports, and even conflicting advice from medical professionals. The decision really comes down to deciding: are the risks worth the benefits that HRT can deliver?

Before I discuss these risks and benefits further, it's worth understanding the rather provocative history of HRT.

A quick history of HRT

HRT for menopause has been around longer than you might suspect – since the late 1800s. As early as the 1930s menopausal women were routinely offered extracts of human placenta or oestrogen distilled from the urine of pregnant women in what was later described as 'socialized estrogenicity', whereby the 'estrogen-rich woman gives to the estrogen-poor'.[252]

The drug Premarin, which is made from urine extracted from pregnant mares – don't be too horrified, for years insulin for diabetes was extracted from pig's pancreases – was first marketed in the 1940s. Hormone doses in these early preparations were far in excess (in the order of ten times) of those prescribed today, and modern doses of HRT contain less synthetic hormones than found in some versions of the oral contraceptive pill.

By the mid-1970s it became apparent HRT was not without its risks, and studies showed links between oestrogen therapy and endometrial cancer. This led to the finding that women with a uterus also need progesterone added to the mix to prevent endometrial cancer (women without a uterus because of hysterectomy don't need added progesterone).

In 1972, one of the more lyrical women's health papers ever written appeared in *The Journal of the American Geriatrics Society*, penned by New York gynaecologist Robert Wilson and his wife, a nurse, Thelma Wilson. It claims the oestrogen molecule is by far the most important hormone in the body. 'Estrogen produces the beauty, the allure which attracts the male. This can no more be resisted than the moth can resist the flame. Instead of death there results life – that is why we are here.'[252]

In the paper, the Wilsons describe menopause as 'a galloping catastrophe' and a time of 'slowly foundering sexuality' treatable by the simple transfer of natural oestrogens from one mammal to another. They posit that the timely administration of natural oestrogens plus progesterone to middle-aged women will prevent the climacteric, 'a syndrome that seems unnecessary for most of the women in the civilized world.'

The Wilsons correctly identify many of HRT's positive benefits. Oeostrogen 'will inhibit osteoporosis and thus help to prevent fractures, as long as they continue healthful activities and appropriate diets. Breasts and genital organs will not shrivel.' Although the final line surely reflects the era in which it was published: 'Such women will be much more pleasant to live with and will not become dull and unattractive.'[252]

The 1970s marked the beginning of the sexual revolution and at the same time that younger women were embracing the reproductive freedom begotten by the contraceptive pill, older women were embracing HRT as an elixir of youth, freeing them from hot flashes, sleepless nights and mood swings (and becoming dull and unattractive).

During the 1990s prescriptions for HRT skyrocketed, with US statistics citing up to ninety million women were taking HRT by 1999.[253] While millions embraced HRT, others questioned whether naturally dwindling hormone stores should be viewed as a problem. They resisted the notion that women of a certain age suffered from 'oestrogen deficiency' that needed restoration in order to function as feminine. They pointed towards our Western obsession with youth and beauty as the problem, not ageing ovaries.

Similar debates about HRT can be heard today, but with an extra frisson of fear.

Fear, loathing and women's health studies

In the decades since the 1970s, numerous women's health studies have been conducted to learn about the risks and benefits of HRT.

The Women's Health Initiative (WHI) is a randomised controlled trial designed to examine the effects of HRT on heart attacks, stroke, blood clots, bone fractures, breast, colon and uterine cancer, and overall causes of death. Over 27000 healthy women aged fifty to seventy-nine were enrolled and randomly assigned to receive HRT or placebo.[254]

In 1996 the Million Women Study began recruiting one million UK women aged fifty to sixty-four into a cohort study to research how various reproductive and lifestyle factors, including HRT, affect women's health.[255]

Other studies include the Nurses' Health Study, which has followed the health of several hundred thousand US nurses to see if there is a relationship between medical and lifestyle choices such as the oral contraceptive pill, alcohol use, exercise, cigarette smoking, obesity and, of course, HRT. Thanks to the nurses, we know that a Mediterranean-style diet reduces the risk of colon cancer, and obesity increases the risk of stroke.[256]

The post-menopausal oestrogen/progesterone interventions (PEPI) randomised controlled trial ran from 1987 to 1990 and studied 800 women aged forty-five to sixty-four to learn about the risks and benefits of various HRT regimens. Thanks to PEPI we know HRT increases breast density on a mammogram, which makes it harder to detect breast cancers if they do occur.[257]

The Study of Women's Health Across the Nation (SWAN) is an observational study that has followed over 3000 American women from perimenopause through their transition. SWAN is significant because it has taken into account women's ethnic backgrounds, and found that ethnicity plays a big part in the menopausal transition experience.[258]

In July 2017, the North American Menopause Society (NAMS) released a position statement that came about after society members reviewed decades of data amassed from millions of women to see the effects of HRT. The extraordinary list of women's health issues considered included cancers, heart disease, diabetes, mood, osteoporosis and fracture prevention, hot flashes, musculoskeletal and joints, and on and on. NAMS concluded that the benefits of HRT outweigh the risks for healthy women with menopausal symptoms.[251]

There are many other studies I could mention but I don't want to bore you; instead, I want you to appreciate that HRT is actually a well-researched and scrutinised women's health issue. We have very detailed information about the risks and benefits for a wide range of health outcomes.

Why, despite the wealth of knowledge we have available, is there still so much fear and confusion around HRT?

It all comes down to the WHI and the dramatic events that unfolded in 2002 and 2003. I was working at a national breast cancer organisation at the time when news filtered in that stunned us all. WHI announced it had stopped the oestrogen plus progestin arm of the trial because of safety issues. It appeared that combined HRT caused a small increased risk of breast cancer, heart disease, stroke and blood clots.

While researchers and statisticians immediately pointed out that the risks were greatly exaggerated and there were errors in the original paper, media attention was understandably extraordinary. Women on the trial were sent letters telling them to stop, and doctors were inundated with calls from frantic patients. Many doctors advised their patients to come off HRT, and it has been estimated that globally fifty to eighty per cent of women stopped HRT.

In 2003 it was reported combined HRT increased the risk of dementia in postmenopausal women aged sixty-five years and older.[259] The Million Women Study followed with a 2003 report in the *Lancet* claiming use of HRT increased the incidence of breast cancer.[260] I remember the CEO of my organisation spending days fielding calls and media interviews from what can only be described as her 'HRT war room'.

In the fifteen years since the alarm bell rang, studies have continued to gather and analyse data, and our current understanding of the risks and benefits is far more nuanced.

The major problem with the WHI study was that the average age of women entering the trial was sixty-three; only ten per cent of women were younger than fifty-five when they began treatment. We now understand that the effects of HRT vary depending on the age at which it's given. Most women in the WHI were simply too old to be starting HRT safely.

We've since learned that there is a critical window for starting HRT – the window closes within a few years of a woman's last period. HRT can be taken safely, but only if treatment starts within the critical window when women are young; ideally, when symptoms first appear. If older women start treatment decades after their menopause, the risks of HRT do indeed outweigh the benefits.[251]

In other words, timing is everything.

Research has also shown there is no 'one-size-fits-all' approach to HRT. Instead, decisions about the type, dose, formulation, route of administration and duration of use should be based on the unique health risks of each woman, her age or time from menopause, and her goals for therapy. The old blanket advice, 'take the lowest dose for the shortest period of time', has been dropped.

Weighing up the risks and benefits of HRT

A generation of women have missed out on HRT because of fear about developing breast cancer, blood clots or heart disease. Of course, no therapy is without risk, but for perspective let's put your risk of developing breast cancer into context. Within a given year,[249]

♀ if you are taking HRT, you have a 4 in 1000 chance of breast cancer;

♀ if you are *not* taking HRT, you have a 3 in 1000 chance of breast cancer.

Another way to look at it: having more than two standard alcoholic drinks per day or being overweight puts you at a higher risk of developing breast cancer than taking HRT.

You might also find it comforting to know we're getting very good at detecting and treating breast cancer if it does occur. In Australia, ninety per cent of women diagnosed with breast cancer are alive five years later, and if the cancer is limited to the breast, ninety-six per cent will be alive five years after diagnosis.[261]

The risk of having a heart attack related to use of hormone therapy appears to depend on your age.[262] There is no increased risk of heart attacks related to HRT in women who:

♀ start taking HRT less than ten years after their last period, or

♀ were aged fifty to fifty-nine years when they started HRT.

What about the *benefits* of HRT?

Hot flashes. HRT is, hands down, the best evidence-based treatment for hot flashes.

Insomnia. If your sleep disturbances are due to night sweats and/or hot flashes, HRT improves sleep. In women with sleep problems without hot flashes, HRT doesn't always make a difference.[263] John Eden suggests this may be because many women often delay treatment for sleep issues for some years. Thus, even once hot flashes are controlled, insomnia has been established.

Mood disorders. If anxiety and depression are tied up with disrupted sleep patterns due to hot flashes, HRT is likely to help. And as John Eden said to me, all you can do is trial HRT for a few months and see if it improves your mood. If anxiety or depression are the dominant symptoms without hot flashes, then doctors typically recommend a range of treatments such as those outlined in chapter 6.[264]

Brain fog. Once again, if hot flashes wake you up at night, brain fog may clear with HRT. However, the evidence remains inconclusive at best. Some trials of HRT and verbal memory show a benefit, others show no benefit.

Interestingly, a small pilot trial of nine women conducted by Professor Sue Davis suggests that testosterone (usually given to treat low libido) improves verbal learning and memory in post-menopausal women. 'Much of the research on testosterone in women to date has focused on sexual function,' Davis has said, 'but testosterone has widespread effects in women, including, it appears, significant favourable effects on verbal learning and memory.' Professor Davis doesn't recommend that women experiencing brain fog visit their doctor to ask for a script for testosterone because much larger randomised, placebo-controlled trials are necessary. As we'll learn in chapter 10, keeping your brain healthy and your thinking clear also requires attention to good nutrition, physical exercise, adequate sleep, stress reduction and mental stimulation.[265]

Sexual dysfunction (including symptoms such as vaginal dryness) and muscle aches and pains may also improve with HRT.

As John Eden told me, there is no other health condition he knows of where symptoms are simply endured when there is a safe, cheap, effective treatment on hand. 'I see women giving up work because of their menopause,' he said, 'but most of my cancer patients carry on working through their treatments.'

The benefits can perhaps be summarised best by a friend of mine who said, 'It made me feel like me again.' For this woman it wasn't a question of chasing eternal youth, rather, making the informed decision to face the next few decades of her life with mental and physical vigour.

There are various additional risks and benefits that must be weighed up for each woman, for example, a history of breast cancer, gene mutations predisposing them to breast cancer, early menopause or surgical menopause, cardiovascular disease risk factors and so on. There are also plenty of complexities around the combinations of hormones (oestrogen and/or progesterone and/or testosterone), and how you take them (pill, gel, patch, vaginal pessary, micronised, bio-identical, lozenge, etc). Such considerations are well outside the scope of this book, and as the saying goes, please consult a good women's health doctor (not a sales rep for an online store!). Here in Australia, the Jean Hailes organisation is my go-to resource for up-to-date, evidence-based, simple information written for a non-medical-professional audience.

Let's hope this information will allow conversations between women and their health-care providers about initiating, continuing or stopping HRT to be 'evidence-based, and not fear-based'.[251]

Does HRT cause or prevent dementia?

The evidence is very clear that HRT does *not cause* dementia or AD. The most recent large trial of 27 347 women who were followed for eighteen years found deaths from AD and other forms of dementia were significantly *lower* with oestrogen-alone medication than with a placebo.[266]

The fear that HRT caused dementia arose from the results of the Women's Health Initiative Memory Study (WHIMS), which was a sub-group of WHI. For the 4532 women included in the trial, HRT worsened cognitive function, and increased the risk for AD. Despite this trial being of 'gold standard' (it was randomised, double-blind and controlled) there was the same glaring problem with the protocol: women were enrolled at the average age of seventy-two, roughly fifteen to twenty years *after* their menopause, and well beyond the critical window of opportunity in which HRT is of benefit. Unfortunately, WHIMS came to the *incorrect* conclusion that HRT was detrimental to brain health and caused AD. We now understand that HRT increases dementia risk only if it is begun *after* the critical period has closed.[259]

A much smaller study of 428 women has explored the effects of HRT timing on brain health.[267] Women who started HRT during perimenopause scored better on the Mini-Mental State Examination – a test of cognition and attention – compared to women who started HRT after menopause. And women who started HRT 'late' scored worse on the test than women who never used hormone therapy.

The critical window hypothesis is supported by careful studies of the effects of hormone therapy on female rodents. In rats, the perimenopause is a window of opportunity for oestrogen therapy to protect the brain against declines in cognitive function and related neurodegenerative diseases. When oestrogen is administered to middle-aged rats during perimenopause, it improves memory and protects against dementia. When oestrogen is administered to elderly post-menopausal rats after a prolonged period of hormone deprivation, oestrogen loses its neuro-protective power. Some researchers propose that the menopausal transition is an additional 'critical period of brain plasticity', similar to infancy, adolescence and pregnancy, one in which the anti-ageing effects of oestrogen can be harnessed to promote healthy brain ageing in the decades that follow.[268]

In short, HRT may prove to be protective against unhealthy brain ageing if started when menopausal symptoms emerge, and damaging for brain health if started years after menopause. But just to be clear, there is no expert consensus on the use of HRT to *prevent* unhealthy brain ageing or forms of dementia. We know HRT does no harm, but as yet no trials in which HRT has been administered within the critical window have been running long enough to conclude whether or not there is a benefit. Watch this space.

Mind the gap of midlife

Carl Jung wrote, 'The afternoon of human life must also have a significance of its own and cannot merely be a pitiful appendage to life's morning.'[269]

Apart from menopause, we tend to think of midlife as a quiescent period that lies between the turmoil of adolescence and the decline of old age. Yet midlife is when we're at the peak of parenting, decision-making, self-confidence, self-esteem, and our capacity to earn and contribute to the community. Midlife is also when the early warning signs for poor brain and physical health emerge, but when there is still time to delay, minimise or even prevent some of the changes in the biological, psychological and social functioning that typically occur in later life.

Midlife is a unique window of opportunity in which to invest in future-proofing your brain. It's time to stop, take stock and invest in a healthy future. In the words of John F Kennedy, 'The time to repair the roof is when the sun is shining.'

10.

The Ageing Brain

WHEN DOES OLD AGE BEGIN?

We can't seem to make up our minds, and the older we get, the further we move the goalposts marking the last season of our lives.

A 2009 survey of Americans asked participants when they believed someone grew 'old'. Young folks in their twenties believed old age began at sixty. Those under fifty put the threshold closer to seventy, whereas those sixty-five and above said that the average person does not become old until turning seventy-four.[270]

Getting old isn't nearly as bad as people think it will be. Nor is it quite as good.

On the downside, one in four adults aged sixty-five surveyed reported memory loss. One in five had serious illness, were no longer sexually active, or often felt sad or depressed, lonely or had trouble paying bills. One in ten felt like a burden.

On the upside, the same group said they had more time for hobbies, travel and volunteer work, and more financial security. Of all the good things about getting old, the best by far, according to older adults, was being able to spend more time with family members.

One of my boys said to me recently he couldn't imagine me as a little girl and asked how it felt to finally be 'old'. I told him I feel the same now as I did when I was ten. 'Am I old? Certainly not!' was the answer survey respondents gave too. In fact, the older they got, the younger they said they felt. About half of those under thirty said they felt their age. But those who were seventy-five and older? Just thirty-five per cent say they felt 'old'.

The survey results show that as we age we remain on intimate terms with our much younger selves. Similarly, we enter the end of our lifespan with our past woven intimately into our biology. From birth, our neural architecture is shaped by life's ups and downs, the decisions we make, the places where we live, work and learn, the meaning we've derived, and who we love, give life to, and travel with through time. How we spend our early years will determine how we age.

More and more of us are living into old age, and there has never been a better time in which to do so. Our large, clever human brains have bestowed us with modern medicine and tools with which we manage our reproductive health, avoid maternal and neonatal death, vaccinate against disease, prevent pain, treat infection and some cancers, and perform surgery if required. One hundred years ago, women lived barely long enough to see out their fifties. A baby girl born today can expect to live to see out the first decades of the twenty-second century.

We've living longer, but how do our ageing brains fare?

Dementia, memory loss and cognitive decline are robustly related to old age, and AD is one of the leading causes of death globally. So, is the payoff for a longer life memory loss and poor brain health in our final years?

To answer this question, I've looked to two sources: those exceptionally old folks who remain in robust physical and mental health until the very end of their lives, and our evolutionary past.

Over millennia, Mother Nature equipped us to survive and thrive in the wild. Our brains evolved such that from the womb to the tomb we're required to move, eat well, sleep, immerse ourselves in nature, avoid stress, love and befriend, and seek meaning. These bottom-up, outside-in and top-down requirements neatly match the everyday life prescriptions followed by the world's longest-living people.

Prevention is our best defence and the research on dementia is clear. Those of us who lead mentally, socially and physically stimulating lives have reduced risk of age-related brain disease. If we live as close as possible to how Mother Nature intended, while reaping the rewards of our modern health care, there is every chance we can add not only years to our lives, but life to our years.

Uncovering the secrets of exceptional longevity

On 21 February 1875, one year before Alexander Graham Bell filed his patent for the telephone, a baby girl, Jeanne Louise Calment, was born in Arles, France. She was alive to witness the invention of the aeroplane and the cinema; on a trip to Paris she saw the Eiffel Tower being built and she reported she met Vincent Van Gogh. In 1997, the same year Diana, Princess of Wales died, Calment finally passed away. She was 122 years and 164 days old. Although blind, almost deaf and confined to a wheelchair, Calment reportedly remained spirited and 'alert as a hummingbird' till the end. The French called her *la doyenne de l'humanité* (the elder of humankind) and she still holds the record for the world's longest-ever living human.[271]

In April 2017, Emma Martina Luigia Morano of Vercelli, Italy, died aged 117. Born in November 1899, Morano was the last known living person who was born in the 1800s. According to the *Guinness Book of Records*, Morano followed the same extraordinary diet for around ninety years: three eggs per day (two raw, one cooked), fresh Italian pasta and a dish of raw meat. The current longevity crown belongs to Japanese centenarian Nabi Tajima, who was born in August 1900 on Kikaijima, a remote island off the southern coast of Japan.

Once rare as diamonds, the oldest of the old are the fastest-growing sector of our global population. If you were born in 1900 the odds of living till age 100 were less than one in a million, and few people lived long enough to see out the 1950s. For girls born into wealthy countries today, the odds of blowing out 100 candles on a cake are roughly one in fifty.

When asked her secret to old age, Jeanne Calment attributed her longevity to immunity to stress and a good attitude. 'I wasn't afraid of anything. I was often reproached for that,' she said. 'I took pleasure when I could, I acted clearly and morally and without regret. I'm very lucky.' Calment reportedly ate more than two pounds of chocolate a week, treated her skin with olive oil, rode a bicycle until she was 100, and only quit smoking when she was 117 because she became too proud to ask someone else to light her cigarettes. Known for her wit, she is widely reported as saying, 'I've never had but one wrinkle, and I'm sitting on it.'

Hard work, raw eggs, biking and no regrets. We clamour to learn their secrets, and typically the oldest of the old love to share their long-won wisdom. 'I wait. For death and journalists,' Calment once quipped.

Centenarians certainly provide us with a unique opportunity to uncover the secrets of longevity. And for one group of researchers in Sydney, Australia, exceptionally old folk are providing an insight into successful healthy brain ageing. Charlene Levitan and colleagues at the University of New South Wales (UNSW) Centre for Health Brain Ageing (CHeBA) run the Sydney Centenarian Study, a project that includes over 400 residents from the suburbs of Sydney who are aged over ninety-five.

'Modern medicine has enabled us to add years to our life, but I think it's really important to also add life to our years,' said Levitan to me on the phone. 'Because of this, I'm trying to uncover, through the world of neuroscience and medicine, the keys to successful ageing, so we can all live longer and healthier lives. I'm passionate about recognising the value of the oldest people in our society, the wisdom that we can learn from them that can enrich our society as a whole.'

Centenarians are recruited to the study from Sydney suburbs, chosen to be representative of the Australian population as a whole. 'We have people who are severely demented and people who are extremely high functioning,' says Levitan. 'One of our aims is to try to be inclusive and cover the full continuum of mental and physical function.' Once their age is verified and cross-checked with official records, all participants have their mental, physical, cognitive and social health assessed and, if they're able, they undergo an MRI and blood tests. Finally, they're invited to enrol in the Sydney Brain Bank donation program. 'During the third phase of assessment we conduct an autobiographical interview. The interview adds richness to the study, and I just love the stories and the connection, the time and the patience they show,' says Levitan.

In another longevity project, *National Geographic* writer Dan Buettner famously identified five 'Blue Zones' around the globe where the residents live to exceptional old age. Despite being from very different parts of the world, there are commonalities to the residents' lifestyles. 'Their longevity has nothing to do with brute discipline, diets, exercise programs or supplements,' says Buettner. He believes the longevity of Blue Zones residents is a result of living in the right environment that constantly 'nudges' residents into living healthy lifestyles.[272]

Residents of the Nicoya Peninsula in Costa Rica prioritise friendship and family, and they almost never work extra hours if it means they have to forgo a good party. They also foster *plan de vida* or a reason to live.

In Loma Linda, California, the strong sense of purpose, day of rest, no-smoking policy and healthy diet practices of the local Seventh Day Adventist community have rubbed off on the health of the whole town.

Residents of the mountainous villages of Sardinia, Italy and the Greek island of Ikaria, nap, fast, grow their own food and drink wine daily with friends. It's thought the clean air, warm breezes and rugged terrain of the Mediterranean islands draw locals outdoors to move naturally.

The residents of the Japanese islands of Okinawa, home to the world's longest-living women, are dedicated to family. Okinawans practise *Hara hachi bu*, a reminder to stop eating when they're eighty per cent full; *ikigai*, which roughly translates to 'Why I wake up in the morning', and form *moais*, groups of five friends who remain committed to each other for life.

Buettner has distilled the lifestyle practices of Blue Zones into lessons for longevity. As he says, to make it to 100 you may have to 'win the genetic lottery', but the average person's life expectancy can be increased by moving, prioritising friends, family and social gatherings, eating less, drinking wine and fostering a sense of purpose.

Due to the rarity of extremely old folks, the Sydney Centenarian Study has partnered with a consortium of centenarian research teams from around the globe to pool their resources and data to enable more powerful conclusions to be drawn. Their data supports the Blue Zones observations.

'What is emerging from the global research is that around thirty per cent of longevity is contributed by genetics,' said Levitan. 'The remaining seventy per cent is to do with our lifestyle, which includes a healthy diet, exercise and remaining socially integrated.' One of the strongest themes to emerge is related to the personality traits of resilience, adaptability and optimism. 'Most of our centenarians will report optimism as a life-long personality characteristic,' said Levitan.

Are the exceptionally old also exceptionally happy and healthy?

My mother often says to me there's no way she'd want to live to 100. And she may have a point. It's all well and good following longevity principles in an attempt to add years to your life, but what about the life *during* those years?

'There is certainly a myth out there that the older you get, the sicker you become,' says Levitan, who has found that centenarians usually remain in remarkably good health until extreme old age, with illness compressed into the very end of life. Similarly, Blue Zones residents are unique not only because of their extended lifespan but their long years lived free of disease and disability – what's known as a long 'health-span'.

A *British Journal of Psychiatry* report of Jeanne Louise Calment's health at age 118 is another example. 'The subject's performance on tests of verbal memory and language fluency is comparable to that of persons with the same level of education in their eighties and nineties. Frontal lobe functions are relatively spared and there is no evidence of depressive symptomatology or other functional illness,' writes Karen Ritchie, a neurologist who examined Calment. Ritchie points out that 'it may be unreasonable to generalise from a single case study', and Calment may be a 'statistical outlier'; however, Calment is actually the norm.[273] As a group, centenarians have a remarkable ability to sidestep the usual diseases and maladies of old age.

Levitan explained to me that researchers have now identified three broad groups of centenarians: Escapers, Delayers and Survivors, so named because of the routes they've taken to avoid the major age-related diseases that kill off their peers.

'Escapers are those very lucky people who have managed to escape illness altogether, and are living till 100 with remarkably strong mental and physical capabilities,' said Levitan. 'Then there are the Delayers, who tend to delay any age-related illness until their late eighties. Finally, the Survivors are those people who have been diagnosed with an age-related disease such as cancer, stroke, heart attack, diabetes, and so on. And yet, remarkably, they've survived.'

Another longevity project, the New England Centenarian Study (NECS) found that for every five centenarians, one was an Escaper, two were Survivors and two were Delayers. Even though men were far less likely to reach 100, they were twice as likely to be Escapers than women. Men and women were equally likely to be Survivors or Delayers.

Male centenarians appear to be healthier than their female counterparts. Regardless of their age, men experience a swifter decline to death, with their poor health compressed into a very short space of time. For women, the trajectory from good health to death is often slower and filled with more doctors' visits and frailty.[274]

In one sense, the extremely old become orphans of time. Extreme old age brings a thinned social landscape with the death of life partners and friends.[275] This picture sounds depressing and lonely, yet there is a paradox: the older you get, the happier you are.

Compared to middle age, extremely old folks' emotional wellbeing, happiness and optimism is, on average, higher. In a paper titled 'The Emotion Paradox in the Aging Brain', Mara Mather, a gerontologist at UC Davis explains that older adults are less physically and emotionally reactive to stress than younger adults. 'When older adults experience interpersonal tensions, they engage less in destructive conflict strategies, such as yelling, arguing or name calling, and generally find tense interpersonal situations less stressful than younger adults do,' writes Mather. Healthy older adults' ability to roll with the punches is likely due to a number of factors, including wisdom, judgement, experience and age-related changes in the brain.[276]

Predicting who will reach 100

Can we predict in advance who will receive a telegram from the Queen? Are centenarians grown-up versions of the exceptionally resilient dandelion children we met in earlier chapters?

I put these questions to Professor Richie Poulton, head of the Dunedin Multidisciplinary Health and Development Study. Remember, the Dunedin Study has closely charted every detail of the lives of over 1000 people born in the mid-1970s. The cohort is now entering middle age, and Poulton believes he already has a fair idea who will be blowing out 100 candles on their cake. 'It is quite obviously evident,' he says.

Poulton and his team have measured the pace of biological ageing in his 1000-strong cohort. Biological ageing is estimated by charting the 'coordinated decline in the integrity of multiple organ systems', including eighteen biomarkers of cardiovascular, metabolic, endocrine, lung, liver, kidney, immune and dental health. Across twelve years, the biomarkers were measured at three time points when the cohort members were aged twenty-six, thirty-two and thirty-eight. Despite being in their forties and still being too young to have age-related disease, clear patterns emerged. 'From ages twenty-six to thirty-eight we see increasing differentiation between groups in terms of their physical health and mental health,' Poulton says. Based on their pace of ageing scores, three groups were identified: an average group who experienced one year of physiological decline per calendar year; a fast-ageing group who experienced more than twice this rate of change, and a slow-ageing group who experienced almost no change at all.

Poulton's team then chose six personal-history characteristics already linked to poor health and mortality: familial longevity, childhood social class, adverse childhood experiences, childhood health, intelligence and self-control. As he writes in a 2017 report in *Aging Cell*, 'Study members with shorter-lived grandparents, who grew up in lower social class homes, who experienced more adverse childhood events, who had poorer childhood health, who scored lower on IQ tests, and who had poorer self-control all showed evidence of accelerated biological ageing during their twenties and thirties.'

'The fast-ageing group is going to enter the second half of their life in bad shape and get worse,' predicts Poulton. 'We need to start looking at ageing younger than you might think, because therapies will need to be delivered by midlife in order to make a difference.' He tells me the great sadness of his life is knowing he won't live long enough to see if his predictions come true. 'I'll be pushing up daisies by then,' he says.[277]

Of course, not all centenarians or slow-agers are alike and personal histories are unique. The NECS team has found their cohort varied widely in years of education (no years to postgraduate), socioeconomic status (very poor to very rich), religion, ethnicity, and patterns of diet (strictly vegetarian to extremely rich in saturated fats).

However, centenarians in Sydney, New England and Okinawa do share a few key characteristics:

- ♀ They're nearly always lean.
- ♀ They rarely smoke (Calment was an exception).
- ♀ They're better able to buffer stress than most people.
- ♀ Women have a history of bearing children after the age of thirty-five or even forty years.
- ♀ They score low on personality traits of neuroticism, and high on optimism and purpose.

Exceptional longevity clearly runs in families – the children and siblings of centenarians are healthier, have a more favourable 'biological signature', and they age slower. Tellingly, Jeanne Calment's brother François lived till the age of ninety-seven, but as she put it: 'God didn't want there to be two hundred-year-olds in the same family, so it fell to me.'[271]

Does this mean that extreme longevity is genetic?

'Not at all,' say members of the Okinawan Centenarian Study team, also part of the global consortium. 'We believe the Okinawans have both genetic and non-genetic longevity advantages – the best combination – the dietary habits, the physical activity, the psychological and social aspects, all play an important role in Okinawan longevity.'[278]

It turns out that we all have the genetic capability to live to at least our eighties. As the NECS team explains, this makes sense in the context of the study of Seventh Day Adventists in Loma Linda who live eight to ten years longer than the average

American in neighbouring towns. As a group, they tend to be physically fit, vegetarian non-smokers who spend a lot of time with their families and with their church group. Plenty of Americans make nearly the opposite health choices and as a consequence die younger. 'What the Seventh Day Adventist results also show us is that the average American has the genes to reach their mid late eighties, they just need to take very good care of themselves with proper lifestyle choices,' says the NECS team.[279]

Why do women live longer than men?

All over the world, women live longer than men. In Australia in 2016, the median age at death was 85.0 years for women and 78.9 years for men. The gender gap grows with age: among centenarians worldwide, women outnumber men nine to one. The female advantage is not restricted to humans, as for other species, from honeybees to orca whales to rodents, females outlive males.[280, 281]

The size of the gender gap in longevity has always ebbed and flowed. Mortality before modernity was influenced by wars, infection and death during childbirth. In nineteenth century Europe, life expectancy was less than forty years and longevity of men and women was generally very similar. High female mortality due to pregnancy and childbirth corresponded to a high male mortality from causes related to work, accidental injury or war (both sexes succumbed to infection and disease in equal numbers). The greatest gap was seen during the middle decades of the twentieth century. For example, in the UK in the 1970s the average life expectancy for men was about seven years less than for women. The men who died before their time in the 1970s grew up in the early decades of the twentieth century, when most young men smoked and drank, went to war and worked in physically stressful jobs. Such men became the 'carriers' of excess mortality determined by their misspent youth.

Nowadays, teenagers and young men are three times more likely than young women to die by accidents (usually in a car), suicide, drowning and violence. These rates ensure that by age twenty-five more women are alive than men. In middle age men are still more likely to die in car accidents or from suicide, but illnesses related to smoking, alcohol and poor diet start to emerge, with death from heart disease being the main cause of the gender gap. For men, the risk of heart disease begins in their forties. For women, it doesn't start to increase until after menopause. By late life, men are more likely than women to die from heart disease, cancer and diabetes. Of course, women are not immortal, and we lead the statistics in death from dementia, chronic lower respiratory (lung) disease, cerebrovascular disease, influenza and pneumonia.[281]

The past few decades have seen the gap close. Harvard scientist Thomas Perls, who heads up NECS and the Long Life Family Study (LLFS), suggests it's primarily the reduction in male mortality, as opposed to an increase in female mortality, that is closing the gap. He adds, 'In general, the higher a nation's level of social and economic development, the greater the life expectancy for both men and women and the greater the convergence in the two figures.'

The life experiences and circumstances of women who are now in their eighties and nineties were very different from those of their daughters and granddaughters. Each generation 'carries' their lifestyle load of risk forward.

Only time will tell if girls and boys born today reach 'equality' in mortality.

The influence of biological sex on the lifespan

The secret to longevity is actually quite simple: avoid dying young! Do women live longer because we pay closer attention to Blue Zones lifestyle advice or because we make more visits to the doctor, thereby avoiding early death?

Probably not. As mentioned, elderly women often spend their extra few years of life in poor health, and female non-human species generally outlive their male counterparts, so it's doubtful whether we can attribute healthy lifestyle practices to the gender gap.

Clearly, men and women differ genetically, and one theory posits that the female 'backup' X chromosome provides a survival advantage. Men, in contrast, have only one X chromosome, so they cannot rely on a backup if a gene on the X chromosome is defective.

Another theory implicates mitochondria, which exist in almost all animal cells and convert our food into the energy that powers the body. Genetic variation in mitochondria reliably predicts life expectancy in males, but not in females. We receive copies of genes from both parents, except for mitochondrial genes that come only from our mother. It's possible natural selection, which is evolution's 'quality control process', only screens the quality of mitochondrial genes in females, so the mutations related to ageing are carried by males.[282]

Finally, longevity in women might be advantageous for a rather warm and fuzzy reason: grandmothers! Earlier in the book we saw that menopausal orcas contribute to the survival of young whales by guiding the pod to hunting grounds, and a similar theory proposes that human matriarchs confer the same survival benefits through the practice known as 'alloparenting'.

The cute but contentious 'grandmother hypothesis' was first proposed in the 1980s, when anthropologist Kristen Hawkes spent time with the Hadza hunter–gather communities in Tanzania. She noticed that when grandmothers were involved in supporting their daughters by babysitting and gathering food, the grandchildren and the entire tribe were healthier and lived longer. Hawkes took this idea one step further and claimed that grandmothers provide the foundation for human social connection, pair bonding and evolution of bigger brains. Hawkes has since watered down her original hypothesis based on mathematical modelling of human populations, but still claims, 'Grandmothers make us human'.

The influence of reproductive history on the lifespan

Your reproductive history includes the length of time from your menarche to menopause, number of pregnancies, your age at your first and last pregnancies, and duration of breastfeeding. This history reflects your cumulative exposure to sex hormones, and your 'exposure' to parenting, which coalesce to influence both lifespan and health-span in some surprising ways.

For example, the older you are when you give birth to your *last* child, the longer you'll live, a phenomenon first noticed in centenarian women – a remarkable number of whom gave birth to babies late in life. According to the LLFS, women who give birth to a child *after* the age of forty have four times greater odds of reaching 100 compared to women who have their last child *before* the age of forty. And women who have their last child after the age of thirty-three years have twice the odds of exceptional longevity compared to women who have their last child before age twenty-nine.[283]

The age at which you give birth to your *first* baby matters too. Time and time again, studies have found that women who give birth in their teens experience worse health as they age, and they die younger than women who delay their first pregnancy. Sadly, socioeconomic status contributes to this statistic. Teenage mothers are more likely to have grown up in disadvantaged households than women who delay their first pregnancy, and by virtue of raising a child from a young age, they're less likely to stay in education and more likely to continue the cycle of disadvantage.[284]

Over the years, there have been conflicting reports on whether the *number* of children you have influences lifespan. It turns out that the relationship between motherhood and mortality follows a J-shaped curve. If, like me, you're partial to a glass of red wine, you may be familiar with the 'J-shaped' curve for alcohol consumption and health, whereby a glass or two of wine a day is more beneficial for health than nothing, or drinking to excess. Like glasses of wine, having two or three children is better for your health and longevity than remaining childless, or giving birth to four or more.[284]

Finally, having short birth intervals between your children (less than eighteen months apart or having twins or triplets) is linked to worse health, increased prescriptions for antidepressants (hardly a surprise), and increased mortality than if you space your children out by two to three years. Researchers state that the 'emotional, psychological and social strains of raising multiple children' has 'adverse long-term effects on parental health.'[285] I concur: the stresses and strains of having two boys under two with no extended family on hand quickly took its toll on my mental health. I only hope that the fact I snuck my two in just after the magic age of thirty-three will somehow counterbalance the strain!

Interestingly, the J-shaped relationship between health and number of children, and birth spacing is also present for fathers.

The more children men have, the higher their risk of death from alcohol-related disease, heart disease and accidents. While it might be tempting to say children drive men (and women) to drink (or justify their glasses of wine), there's no evidence the relationship between your children and your health is causal; instead, a *correlation* exists.

It remains to be seen whether cumulative exposure to oestrogen, or pregnancy per se contribute to longevity. However, broadly speaking, like an apple a day, oestrogen protects and keeps the doctor away.

Certainly, there is data showing that having babies and breastfeeding them protects against some cancers, especially breast and ovarian cancer. The protective effect is strongest if you have children before the age of thirty and breastfeed them for a year or more. It's thought protection is due to reduced exposure to monthly fluctuations of oestrogen and progesterone, rather than a reduction in overall exposure.

For women who make the decision to take HRT, the results of eighteen years of follow-up on HRT trials should provide reassurance. A report published in *JAMA* in 2017 found 'no long-term increase in all-cause mortality or mortality from specific causes, such as cardiovascular disease or cancer, among women who received hormone replacement therapy (HRT) for five to seven years.'[266] And as we discussed in chapter 9, there is a reduced risk of AD and improved cognition if you start using HRT within the critical window (i.e. beginning when menopausal symptoms emerge, not years later). Earlier age at menarche, later age at last pregnancy and use of the pill also protect against cognitive decline in later life.

It's important to note that most data on reproductive history, hormonal status and longevity are crunched from large population-based studies, often from Scandinavian countries where the government keeps particularly detailed health records. For example, the birth-spacing finding came from Norway, where researchers were able to gather complete health histories for all women and men ever born and living in the country after 1935. Similarly, the data on family size come from the Swedish population register for all people born and living in the country between 1932 and 1960.

We have a tendency to turn 'research' into 'me-search' and view the data through our own life lens. So it's important to keep in mind that the benefits and harms I'm mentioning are based on averages across large populations, and not always directly applicable to each of us.

Thomas Perls agrees: 'This does not mean women should wait to have children at older ages in order to improve their own chances of living longer. The age at last childbirth can be a rate-of-aging indicator. The natural ability to have a child at an older age likely indicates that a woman's reproductive system is aging slowly, and therefore so is the rest of her body.'[286] So, if you're in your teens or twenties, it's probably unwise to apply data on longevity to your future family planning.

Is dementia a women's brain health problem?

More women than men develop AD or other dementias. There are a number of potential biological and social reasons for this fact.

One prevailing view is simply that, on average, women live longer than men, and getting older is the greatest risk factor for AD.

A related reason is men's 'survival bias'. Men who live to old age tend to be much healthier than women of the same age and therefore have lesser risks of developing AD.

Another well-known genetic risk factor for AD is the gene APOE-e4. A 2017 meta-analysis of nearly 58 000 people found that women with particular versions of APOE-e4 may be more likely to develop AD than men with the same version of the gene, but only between the ages of sixty-five and seventy-five years.[287]

One final reason often given to account for the sex difference in risk is low education in women. The more years of schooling you receive, the lower your risk of developing AD, and the simple fact women born before the 1950s typically completed fewer years of education than men might have rendered their brains more vulnerable to the disease in old age.[288]

In September 2017 the Australian Bureau of Statistics (ABS) released a report stating that dementia is the leading cause of death among Australian women. For men, dementia took out number two spot, right behind heart disease. The ABS warns that as treatments for heart disease improve, and men live longer, healthier lives, dementia will likely surpass heart disease as the leading cause of death for men too.[289]

We are privileged to live in a world where life expectancy is increasing; and the ageing population, which worries so many people, is actually one of humanity's greatest achievements. The cost of our longevity is that dementia has become humanity's brain health problem.

Dementia – humanity's brain health problem

The 2015 World Alzheimer Report on the global impact of dementia states there are over 9.9 million new cases of dementia each year worldwide, which implies one new case every 3.2 seconds. In 2015, the estimated number of people living with dementia was 22.9 million in Asia, 10.5 million in Europe, 4 million in Africa, and 9.4 million in the Americas. As baby boomers reach older age, numbers are set to double every twenty years.[290]

The statistics made for disturbing reading and a 2015 WHO report on dementia sums up how many of us feel: 'Dementia is highly stigmatised and universally feared. It is often perceived as a normal part of ageing, and that no actions can be taken to prevent or treat it.'[291]

Although stats vary by country, your absolute risk is probably not as high as you fear. In the UK, about two in 100 (two per cent) of people aged sixty-five to sixty-nine have dementia; this figure rises to one in five (twenty per cent) for those aged eighty-five to eighty-nine. The majority of centenarian studies report rates of dementia in the extremely old as sitting somewhere between forty-five and sixty-five per cent, with the Sydney Centenarian Study rates consistent with this finding. On the upside, eighty per cent of people in their eighties and nearly half of centenarians remain dementia free.

Take heart: contrary to popular belief, dementia is *not* a natural or inevitable consequence of ageing. Dementia is a disease, and while there is no cure, there are steps you can take to tip the brain health scales in your favour.

In late 2015 an international team pooled data from 323 studies including over 5000 people and ninety-three factors thought to influence risk for AD, many of which also increase the risk for cardiovascular disease. A total of nine modifiable harms were found to cause sixty-six per cent of AD cases globally. The most significant harm was heavy smoking, whereas a healthy diet was protective.

For men and women the nine modifiable risk factors included: being obese, smoking, carotid atherosclerosis (hardening of the arteries), Type 2 diabetes, low education, high total homocysteine level, depression, high blood pressure and frailty.

For women, oestrogen therapy (contraceptive pill use or HRT) protected against AD.

The paper concluded with a startling but heartening statement: two in three AD cases worldwide are preventable.[292]

What is dementia? How does it differ from Alzheimer's disease?

Dementia is an umbrella term used to describe the symptoms of a large group of illnesses that cause a progressive decline in a person's functioning. There are over 100 diseases that cause dementia symptoms including AD, frontotemporal dementia (FTD), vascular dementia, Parkinson's disease, dementia with Lewy bodies, Huntington's disease, alcohol-related dementia (Korsakoff's syndrome) and Creutzfeldt-Jakob disease. AD is the most common form of dementia and accounts for fifty to seventy per cent of all cases, which is why the two terms are often used interchangeably.[293]

Early signs of dementia are subtle and vague. Symptoms may include:

♀ Progressive and frequent memory loss.
♀ Confusion.
♀ Personality change.
♀ Apathy and withdrawal.
♀ Anger and aggression.
♀ Loss of ability to perform everyday tasks.

Clearly these symptoms are common for a number of conditions such as vitamin and hormone deficiencies, depression, infections and brain tumours, and, as we discussed in the last chapter, menopause. Therefore, it's essential that a medical diagnosis is obtained at an early stage when symptoms first appear, to ensure that a person who has a treatable condition is diagnosed and managed correctly.

Memory loss with ageing is normal

One of the main symptoms of dementia is memory loss, but as Dementia Australia points out, there is a difference between forgetfulness as a normal part of ageing and as a symptom of dementia, which is a disease. People with dementia show *persistent* and *progressive* loss of memory to the point where it interferes with their ability to carry out normal daily tasks.[248]

Another type of memory loss usually experienced with ageing is mild cognitive impairment (MCI). Typical complaints from someone with MCI include having trouble remembering names of people they met recently, remembering the flow of a conversation, and a greater tendency to misplace things. However, such people are able to function independently and do not show other signs of dementia, such as personality change, confusion, impaired reasoning or judgement.[293]

It's important to realise that even the youngest, fittest and most alert of us forget things from time to time. This is perfectly normal. So those 'tip-of-my-tongue' moments you may have experienced are pretty normal, and not necessarily a sign of dementia. As I said in chapter 9, there is a difference between normal forgetfulness and dementia. It's standard practice to lose your car keys. You only need to worry if you find them then fail to know what they're used for.

We all have a very human tendency to pay attention to moments of forgetfulness and worry more about them as we get older. And sometimes we seek out instances that confirm our greatest fears. For example, recently I've experienced a few more 'senior moments' than usual. Words have been on the tip of my tongue, and I've had instances of walking into a room then wondering what I was there to do. On reflection, I noticed that my 'forgetfulness' emerged about three weeks ago, precisely at the same point in time I started researching and writing about dementia. A prime example of confirmation bias!

Stuck in the moment with dementia

We tend to focus on memory loss as the cardinal sign of dementia. However, people with dementia not only lose their ability to remember the past but also to imagine the future. Muireann Irish is an associate professor of neuroscience at the University of Sydney. Irish and her team are interested in how the brain systems underlying cognitive processes such as memory, imagination and social cognition are damaged in dementia.

As a student at Trinity College in Dublin, Irish famously found that playing soothing music, in particular Vivaldi's 'Spring' movement from 'The Four Seasons', enhanced autobiographical memory recall in people with AD. Probing the memories of people's lives by asking them to recount stories of their school days, weddings, births of their children, a recent holiday or funerals is a common method to assess memory loss.[294]

When listening to Vivaldi versus silence, the AD patients became more relaxed and less agitated, and the release of stress somehow enabled them to recollect and retrieve their memories. 'When we looked at the mechanisms by which music enhanced autobiographical memory, it was not due to a change in attention or arousal,' Irish tells me during a phone call. 'It was due to a reduction in their anxiety.'

As Irish explained to me, most of us consider daydreaming to be an 'idle pursuit', not an important and fruitful brain function that impacts our sense of self, wellbeing and social cognition. 'The fact we've evolved to have sophisticated brain networks that enable us to daydream suggests it has to have some evolutionary adaptive value,' she says. 'Spontaneous mind wandering can give rise to great feats of creativity, new innovations, and people being more socially empathetic.'

Irish described to me a recent study in which she invited healthy young people and patients with dementia to visit her lab, and asked them to watch a series of brightly coloured shapes presented on a screen (a decidedly boring task). At various intervals people were asked what they were thinking about. Invariably, healthy young people replied with fairly complex stories such as how the yellow shape made them think of the sun and sand on their last island beach holiday and the fabulous meal they ate, which in turn reminded them they needed to shop for groceries for dinner that evening. 'They can't help but transport themselves away from the boring task,' said Irish.

For people with dementia, their responses lacked depth and imagination as if they found it difficult to let their minds wander. 'They almost get stuck, in a concrete way, on the stimulus in front of them. "It was a nice yellow triangle" might be a typical response,' she said.

'For people with dementia, the world is anchored in the present. Their ability to remember the past gradually erodes, with only small islands or pockets of memories remaining,' she said. 'Losing the ability to recollect key events from the past strips us of our sense of identity as we cannot recall evocative and defining life events that have shaped us as individuals. While dementia patients do possess a future, it is out of reach as they are unable to envisage and look forward to upcoming events.'

Irish's work is important because it shows that dementia is not just about 'loss of memory' but loss of our very human capacity to daydream and connect not only with our past but with our sense of self and our future.

Taking a closer look at the ageing brain

As we age, our brains shrink in volume and our ventricles (fluid-filled spaces inside the brain) enlarge. From university age onwards we lose roughly 0.2 per cent of our brain weight per year, and the pace picks up to about 0.5 per cent a year when we reach our seventies. So even the healthiest ninety-year-old's brain won't look the same as a millennial's brain.

Surprisingly, 'healthy' shrinkage is not caused by death of cells, rather a loss of rich connectivity between neurons. If you happen upon a microscope and a thin slice of ageing human cortex, you'll notice that elderly neurons look rather like deciduous trees in winter. They're missing their lush foliage as the density of their dendritic arbour shrinks and they retract neurites and spines.

The traditional view that we lose thousands of brain cells every day is wrong. Although the evidence is mixed, perhaps the most surprising finding of the last twenty years – adult human neurogenesis – is that not only are you *not* losing brain cells, you may be gaining them instead.

At the autopsy table, the brain of a patient with AD will look like an extreme version of an elderly brain. The *sulci*, or folds of cortex, will be gaping wide, ventricles will be enlarged and subcortical structures such as the hippocampus will be shrunken. But AD is not an extreme form of ageing – it is a disease and, as such, has a pathological fingerprint.

While the brains of people with AD can be imaged using MRI, a firm diagnosis can only be made at autopsy by viewing the thin sections of brain under a microscope: AD is confirmed by the presence of two proteins in the brain, known as amyloid and tau. Amyloid forms sticky patches or 'plaques' of dense material *outside* neurons. Plaques are often surrounded by dead and dying neurons, swollen axons and dendrites, astrocytes and microglia (a marker of inflammation). If you zoom a microscope lens in further, you'll see twisted filaments of tau, which aggregate *inside* surviving neurons.

How amyloid plaques and tau tangles interact to cause AD symptoms remains a puzzle. Typically, as AD progresses, amyloid and tau deposits spread through the brain, although, curiously, the pathology of the disease does not always correlate with symptoms. For example, you could have very mild symptoms but extensive amyloid accumulation and cell death, or vice versa. One risk factor for the formation of amyloid plaques is a variation of the gene APOE-e4. However, the presence of the gene variation is not itself predictive or diagnostic of AD. Only forty per cent of people with AD carry the gene, and many carriers never go on to develop the disease.

This conundrum has led some researchers to suggest that amyloid is *necessary but not sufficient* for AD. One working hypothesis is that once amyloid appears on the scene, tau accelerates the damage it causes. A commonly used analogy is that amyloid represents the 'bullet' and tau is the 'gun'.[295]

Despite evidence that amyloid accumulation triggers the AD 'cascade', a cure remains elusive. Trials of vaccines and treatments protect against amyloid, once so promising in rodents and primates, have failed in humans.

Underlying the changes in this devastating disease are at least four related biological processes: inflammation, oxidation, glucose and lipid dysregulation – well-known markers of lifestyle disease. While a cure for those already suffering AD continues to elude, and the mechanisms leading to the cascade of pathology are debated, most researchers believe that up to two in three dementia cases can be prevented by lifestyle change.

Proof of principle – using lifestyle change to slow disease

'We're all dealt our unique genetic deck of cards at conception. What matters is how we choose to play our hand.' These wise words were spoken by Professor Tony Hannan, head of the Epigenetics and Neural Plasticity Laboratory at the Florey Institute in Melbourne. Hannan's focus is on understanding how genes (nature) and the environment (nurture) contribute to brain health and to specific brain disorders. 'We're trying to work out a little more about the complex interactions between genes and the environment, and how this translates into susceptibility to neurological and psychiatric conditions.'

Hannan and I first met in Oxford, where he was a postdoc working a few doors along the hall from my PhD lab. He was also delving into the new frontier of nature, nurture and brain plasticity research alongside renowned neurobiologist Colin Blakemore. During this time Hannan worked with mice that had the human gene for Huntington's disease (HD) embedded into their DNA. In humans, HD is a brain disease passed down from parent to child that causes uncontrollable dance-like or jerking movements (chorea), dementia and depression. 'Up until that point, Huntington's was considered to be 100 per cent genetically determined,' he reminded me when we caught up recently, 'but we delayed the onset of the disease with environmental enrichment.'

Compared to their cousins in the wild, lab animals live rather minimalist, unstimulating lives with basic access to food, water and nesting material. Animals in the wild survive by foraging for food and those most adept at outsmarting their predators and competing for resources thrive. It's reasonable to consider laboratory animals as 'couch potatoes' that, compared to rodents in the wild, have sedentary lives with little cognitive challenge.[296]

To simulate life in the wild, Hannan split his HD mice into two groups. Half maintained their couch-potato existence, and half were moved to live in environmentally enriched conditions with access to tunnels, ladders, blocks, mazes and running wheels. 'We discovered that giving this increased sensory and cognitive stimulation and physical exercise delayed the onset of Huntington's disease in mice,' says Hannan. His startling discovery was the first to demonstrate the benefits of enriching experiences on the progress of HD, once thought to be 'the epitome of genetic brain diseases'.

Hannan points out that environmental enrichment in lab animals is roughly equivalent to education in humans. Overwhelmingly the evidence shows that people who attend university undergo less cognitive decline in older age, and are less likely to develop AD than people with fewer years of education. The evidence also points towards certain kinds of challenging jobs (e.g. air traffic controller, financial analyst, doctor) as having the potential to enhance and protect the brain. One study analysed 4182 retirees who'd been doing the same type of work for roughly twenty-five years before they retired. The mental requirements of each job (e.g. analysing data, developing objectives and strategies, making decisions, solving problems, evaluating information and thinking creatively) were assessed alongside each retiree's cognitive health and memory.[297]

Retirees who had worked in jobs with greater mental demands were more likely to have better memories before they retired, *and* more likely to have slower declines in memory after retiring than people who had worked in jobs with fewer mental demands. Work, education or any type of intellectual enrichment that involves a lot of thinking, analysing, problem solving, creativity and other complex mental processing helps build 'cognitive reserve'.

Cognitive reserve refers to the brain's resilience or ability to cope despite damage or degeneration. Professor Yaakov Stern, one of the earliest proponents of the notion, explains, 'In people with a high degree of cognitive reserve, AD pathology will still occur, but people are somehow able to compensate for that damage. Some won't ever be diagnosed with Alzheimer's because they don't present any symptoms,' says Stern. 'Some individuals have a greater number of neurons and synapses, and somehow those extra structures provide a level of protection.'[298]

So where does that leave you if you're not a university-educated air traffic controller with a side gig in medicine? Is it ever too late to build cognitive reserve?

Thankfully, the answer is 'no'. Cognitive decline is not inevitable, because intellectual enrichment goes beyond the work people do. A 2014 Mayo Clinic report found that engagement in cognitively stimulating activities two or three times a week after the age of sixty-five, such as reading books and magazines, playing games or music, artistic activities, craft, social activities and computer activities, all help. Engaging in these activities two or three times a week during mid- and later life may help delay the onset of dementia and tip the scales in your favour.[299]

Hannan's discovery was published in the journal *Nature* in 2000 and paved the way for hundreds of studies extolling the virtues of exercise and cognitive challenge to enhance neuroplasticity, and prevent or treat brain disease and injury. He hopes discoveries in the field of neuroplasticity will inspire each of us to choose to protect our brains from the relentless weathering of ageing and disease.

How to nurture a healthy brain for life

Our human ancestors likely evolved facing similar survival challenges to other species. Whereas the need to acquire food was a major day-to-day challenge during much of our evolutionary history, today we live with a constant oversupply of food. Instead, the intellectual demands of modern life centre on the sedentary tasks of work and education. 'Regular intellectual challenges are critical for brain development and a successful career, and recent findings suggest that intermittent exercise and energy restriction can further enhance and then sustain the functional capabilities of the brain during ageing,' writes Mark P Mattson in *Ageing Brain Reviews*. Rather like an animal in the wild, our intellect evolved to function optimally when we're motivated towards a goal, slightly hungry and on the run, a state Mattson likens to 'Hunger Games' – bolstered brainpower.[300]

In a 2017 *Trends in Neurosciences* paper, University of Arizona researchers David Raichlen and Gene Alexander support Mattson's case that our brains are a product of our evolutionary past. They argue that as humans transitioned from a relatively sedentary apelike existence to a more physically demanding hunter–gatherer lifestyle, starting around two million years ago, we began to engage in complex foraging tasks that were simultaneously physically and mentally demanding, and that may explain how moving and thinking came to be so connected.[301]

The evidence from modern science and ancient wisdom is clear: how we eat, move, sleep, form relationships and find meaning is intimately connected to how our brains grow, think, feel and, ultimately, age.

The best exercise for your brain is physical exercise

Our brains and nervous systems evolved to move us around, sense and interact with the world. Human cognitive prowess and intellect evolved while we were on foot. When faced with inactivity, as is common in our modern-day lives, our brains respond by reducing capacity for neuroplasticity and, as a consequence, brain ageing speeds up.

We have rock-solid evidence that exercise improves mood and reduces risk for age-related brain disease. A 2013 review of twenty-four randomised control trials and twenty-one prospective cohort studies calculated that at least *one in seven cases of AD could be prevented if everyone who is currently inactive took up exercise.*[302]

What type of physical exercise is best?

Jeanne Calment never attended an aerobics class or lifted weights; instead, she rode her bike until she was 100, and lived in a second-storey apartment with no lift until she was 110. People living in Blue Zones don't run marathons, wear Fitbits or join CrossFit gyms. Instead, they live in environments that constantly 'nudge' them into moving without thinking about it. Bike to the grocery store, gather food from the garden, sweep leaves instead of using leaf-blowers, stand instead of sit, swim in the sea, walk to work. Simply moving our bodies throughout our day, instead of exercising to 'get fit' or 'lose weight', is the best way we know to keep our *brains* fit and well.

Eat real food, not too much, mostly plants

Our ancestors and their smart brains were trotting across the landscape hunting, fishing and foraging for food. We evolved to eat food from the rivers, forest and sky. We are also adaptable, and the many versions of a 'healthy diet' vary by country and culture (and, today, by social media platform). What sets apart those who live the longest is not the minutiae of their diet and balance of nutrients gained from fats, protein or carbohydrates, but the absence of refined processed foods.

Evidence from epidemiological studies such as the Blue Zones and clinical trials strongly implicates a Mediterranean-style diet in slowing brain ageing. And most recently a clinical trial in Australia proved successful in treating depression by encouraging young people with depression to increase their consumption of vegetables, fruits, wholegrains, legumes, fish, lean red meats, olive oil and nuts, while reducing their consumption of unhealthy 'extras': foods such as sweets, refined cereals, fried food, fast food, processed meats and sugary drinks.[303]

When we eat we're consuming not only nutrients but energy in the form of calories. Researchers, such as the Dunedin Study team, are now unravelling the relationships among calories, lifespan, health-span and cognitive health. Calorie restriction (eating less) and intermittent fasting (fasting on and off) increase longevity in all species thus far observed, from yeast to rodents to primates – and it's assumed the same is true for us. This notion ties back to the 'Hunger Games' concept whereby our brains evolved to function most optimally when we're hungry and looking for food.[304] Eating less benefits our glucose control and cholesterol, and may produce mild neuronal stress which engages signalling pathways that improve the ability of the brain to resist ageing.

Dietary advice for brain health can be summed up by Michael Pollan's famous adage, 'Eat real food, not too much, mostly plants.'[305]

Get more sleep

As earthlings, our biological rhythms are determined by the rising and setting of the sun. Our sleep patterns, hormone release, blood pressure and body temperature, ebb and flow in sync with day and night.

Modern-day life with its artificial lighting late at night, alarm clocks, shift work, iPhones in bed and jetlag is very good at interfering with our natural sleep patterns. As a basic biological function, sleep is overlooked and under-appreciated, and globally modern humans are chronically sleep deprived. Sleep deprivation (even a few hours a night) impacts cognition, mood, memory and learning, and long-term sleep deprivation leads to chronic disease including depression, diabetes and cardiovascular disease, all risk factors for developing dementia.

A good night's sleep every night should be a priority, not a luxury. My personal daily indulgence – a short afternoon nap – consolidates memory, sparks creativity and smooths rough emotional edges, giving greater control over thoughts and feelings.

Challenge your mind

Lab mice kept in bare cages with no toys or novel environments to explore show greater rates of age-related cognitive decline compared to their counterparts kept in enriched environments full of toys, tunnels and mazes. As we've discussed, humans are no different.

People who stay mentally engaged in life and who constantly challenge themselves to step out of their comfort zones have reduced risk of age-related cognitive decline and dementia.

Children have a natural tendency to run and play, whereas adults tend to take life more seriously. We don't lose the need

for novelty and pleasure once we grow up. Game playing –
whether it be video, traditional board games, dancing, or team
or individual sports – has been shown to alleviate boredom,
anxiety, depression, loneliness, despair and even physical
pain. As Charlene Levitan said to me, 'We don't stop playing
and learning because we get old, we grow old because we stop
playing and learning.'

Find your place or moment of calm

Throughout this book, one pervasive theme has been how
stress 'gets under our skin' to influence our mental and physical
health. Not all stress is bad, but chronic or toxic stress, especially
traumatic life events that are out of our control, has deleterious
effects. The key to buffering stress is to find ways to improve
your perceived ability to cope with whatever life throws your
way.

The evidence is mixed as to whether or not stress *causes*
dementia, but it's clear stress hormones alter risk for anxiety,
depression, obesity and cardiovascular disease, which in turn
increase dementia risk.[306]

More has been spoken or written about the practice of
mindfulness meditation in recent years than any other stress-
relief practice. With good reason: paying attention to your
breath, which is a core component of many mindfulness
practices, reduces anxiety and depression, and improves sleep.

Blue Zones people have in place varied daily rituals that
reduce or buffer the impact of stress in their lives. Activities
include prayer, napping and happy hour with friends (I'll add
walking the dog or enjoying a good book to the mix).

Find peace amid the chaos. Find your place or moment of
calm.

Connect with family and friends

After we foraged, caught and hunted our food, we trotted back to our tribe. Being socially connected to other people protects against stress, and because socialising involves many cognitive functions such as thinking, feeling, sensing, reasoning and intuition, friendships contribute to cognitive reserve.

Old age brings 'costs of survivorship'. 'We lose people with whom we shared many experiences, who are central to our identities, and who are no longer there to validate – or to question – our memories or accounts. This kind of identity loss also occurs with the death of older generations, as we are pushed up the family ladder and, once at the top, become orphans in time,' writes one researcher.[275]

A 2010 meta-analysis of 148 studies including 300 000 people, who were tracked for nearly eight years after completing surveys of how often they met with family and friends, found that socially connected folks live longer. On the flipside, loneliness was associated with late-life loss of cognition, as well as elevated blood pressure, depression and poor sleep. The startling conclusion of this report was that the influence of social isolation on health and risk of death was comparable to smoking.[307]

Seek out meaning and purpose

With purpose and meaning come positive emotions – love, compassion and appreciation – which counteract stress and support a healthy brain throughout life. Blue Zones residents are members of faith communities and find meaning and purpose through social connection and spirituality. Living a meaningful life seems an unlikely addition to a book about the brain, but 'purpose in life' is a concept in neuroscience that links to robust brain and mind health.

Purpose, defined as the tendency to derive meaning from life's experiences and to possess a sense of intentionality and goal directedness that guides behaviour, can be quantified. A study published in *Archives of General Psychiatry* in 2010 examined the association of purpose in life with risk of AD in more than 900 elderly people living in residential care. During the seven years of follow-up, greater purpose in life was associated with a substantially reduced risk of AD, such that a person with a high score on the purpose in life measure was approximately two and a half times more likely to remain free of AD than a person with a low score.[308]

Have you figured out why you're here? What's your north star? Your *ikigai*? Your *plan de vida*? There are possibly many clever strategies to find the meaning of your life – somewhere in the nexus of passion, skillset, employment opportunity, education and service to others. American psychologist William James said in 1920 that the 'deepest principle in human nature is the craving to be appreciated'.

Recently I've come across a simpler way to determine purpose. Over the years I've taken to the stage with Paul Baldock, a bone biologist at Sydney's Garvan Institute of Medical Research. We're often called on to share our wisdom, purpose and what we've learned on our career paths in science. Baldock has developed a novel formula for every decision he makes whether it be in the research lab, career, or life. He simply asks, 'Is it awesome? Does it help?'

Is it ever too late to hope for change?

In an impressive feat of brain plasticity, an enriching life experience changed Jeanne Calment's brain at age 118.

Calment lived an extraordinary life for a woman of her generation. She attended school until the age of sixteen and graduated with a diploma. At twenty-one she married a wealthy distant cousin and recounted to biographers the details of their active lifestyle within the upper society of Arles, pursuing hobbies such as fencing, cycling, mountaineering, swimming, hunting, playing piano and painting, and going to the opera in Marseilles. 'I had fun; I am having fun,' she said.[271]

When Calment was 118, the neuropsychologist Karen Ritchie visited a number of times over a six-month period to examine Calment and submit her to a battery of neuropsychological tests. Ritchie writes, 'Until this program of testing was commenced J.C. had no contact with the outside world apart from the occasional greeting from medical staff and an annual visit from journalists on the occasion of her birthday. For the last three years she has spent her days alone in her room in her armchair.' According to records, Calment enjoyed contributing to the study by recalling the poems, fables and songs she had learned as a child. 'I don't lack for anything. I have everything I need. I've had a good life. I live in my dreams, in my memories, beautiful memories.'

Brain scans showed atrophy of Calment's cortex, but her overall cognitive performance was, in fact, far better than might have been predicted from the extent of brain loss observed. 'There is no evidence at present of senile dementia ... Executive functions (principally controlled by frontal areas), while having deteriorated from young adult levels, appear to be relatively spared ... This raises the question of whether an initially high level of intellectual ability may have been a protective factor,' writes Ritchie.[273]

Remarkably, over the six-month period that Ritchie conducted the testing program, Calment's test scores *improved*. Her verbal recall, narrative recall, verbal fluency and mathematics scores increased from baseline to match those of the average seventy-five to eighty-year-old. Environmental enrichment by way of social interaction with Ritchie and her team, and intellectual stimulation from the testing program activated the latent plasticity in Calment's exceptionally long-lived brain.

Jeanne Calment no doubt had memories that she didn't share, but there was one secret that she wanted to pass on: 'Always keep your sense of humour. That's what I attribute my long life to. I think I'll die laughing. That's part of my program.'[271]

Acknowledgements

I'M A RESEARCHER BY NATURE. LIBRARIES ARE MY NATURAL habitat, with books and papers the tools of my trade. Even so, writing a book is a long, lonely task that involves a lot of time sitting around staring at a screen – not the heathiest prescription for longevity and brain health! That said, the process has been extraordinarily engaging and purposeful. One of the most beautiful sentiments I came across in my research for this book is that our individual life stories are enmeshed with the life stories of other people – we come from someone and somewhere. A story of 'me' is actually a story of 'we', and thanks must go to all those involved.

To my agent Jeanne Ryckmans, for phoning out of the blue one day to ask me why I'd never written a book, convincing me it might be a good idea, and for injecting dramatic fission and hilarious stories along the way. The book would never have come to fruition without you. Thanks to the Sydney publishing team at Hachette. Especially Sophie Hamley for taking a punt on a one-page chapter outline, and for taking me by hand and answering all my novice questions. To the London team at Orion Books, especially Olivia Morris, your enthusiasm for the project came at the perfect time. And to Chris Kunz and Sophie Mayfield for your warm comments and sympathetic editing of the final manuscript.

To Carol Dean, Brigitte Todd, Michelle Guillemard, Dyani Lewis, Kristy Goodwin, Suzanne Newton, Isiah McKimmie, Ruth Hadfield, Bianca Nogrady and Jocelyn Brewer, the experience was enriched thanks to your editing and manuscript suggestions, professional connections, quotes, publishing advice, friendship and virtual gin.

To the many researchers who gave so willingly and candidly of your time over coffee, lunch, phone and Skype (and at times nearly convinced me to consider lab life again), especially Richie Poulton, Bronwyn Graham, Colin and Sarah Akerman, Dave Grattan, Catherine Lebel, Jessica Mong, Margaret McCarthy, Kathleen Liberty, George Patton, Sarah Romans, Jayashri Kulkarni, Lianne Schmaal, Brendan Zietsch, Sarah Whittle, John Eden, Nicole Gervais, Sue Davis, Sonia Davison, Tony Hannan, Charlene Levitan, Lisa Mundy, Lauren Rosewarne and Muireann Irish. And to the many others I've not met but whose research, books and articles informed and inspired this book; any errors reporting your science are my own.

To my far-flung family, friends and neighbourhood crew, your unending supportive Facebook comments and shared bottles of wine made all the difference.

To my affectionate, loyal and furry co-author, Jasper, for patiently listening to me read every single word of this book out loud. You're truly a woman's best friend.

To Dad, especially, for commenting on every single one of my whingeing Facebook posts how proud you are of me.

To Mum and Vicks. Your stories are here, too.

Finally, to my beautiful boys, Harry and Jamie, and gorgeous husband, Geoff. Guess what? Mum is no longer 'writing her book'! The last year may have stolen my attention and time away from you, but the three of you always have my heart. This book is dedicated to you.

Notes

INTRODUCTION

1. Zucker, I. and A.K. Beery, 'Males still dominate animal studies'. *Nature*, 2010. **465**(7299): p. 690.

2. Clayton, J.A., 'Studying both sexes: a guiding principle for biomedicine'. *FASEB J*, 2016. **30**(2): pp. 519–24.

3. Klein, S.L., et al., 'Opinion: Sex inclusion in basic research drives discovery'. *Proc Natl Acad Sci U S A*, 2015. **112**(17): pp. 5257–8.

4. Beery, A.K. and I. Zucker, 'Sex bias in neuroscience and biomedical research'. *Neurosci Biobehav Rev*, 2011. **35**(3): pp. 565–72.

5. Cahill, L., 'An issue whose time has come'. *J Neurosci Res*, 2017. **95**(1–2): pp. 12–13.

6. Rippon, G., 'Blame the brain: How Neurononsense joined Psychobabble to keep women in their place', in *Lecture to the Royal Institution*. 2016, The Royal Institution: London.

7. Joel, D., et al., 'Sex beyond the genitalia: The human brain mosaic'. *Proc Natl Acad Sci U S A*, 2015. **112**(50): pp. 15468–73.

8. NAPLAN, '2016 NAPLAN National Report'. 2016: Australia.

9. McCarthy, M.M., 'Sex Differences in the Brain.', in *The Scientist*. 2015.

10. Fine, C., *Delusions of Gender. The Real Science Behind Sex Differences*. 2010, London: Icon Books.

11. Eliot, L., *Pink Brain, Blue Brain: How Small Differences Grow Into Troublesome Gaps – And What We Can Do About It*. 2010, New York: Houghton Mifflin Harcourt

12. Green, E.R. and L. Maurer, *The Teaching Transgender Toolkit. A Facilitator's Guide To Increasing Knowledge, Decreasing Prejudice & Building Skills*. 2015, NY: Out for Health & Planned Parenthood of the Southern Finger Lakes.

13. 'Sex and Gender. It's Not a Women's Issue'. *Scientific American*, 2017, Springer Nature: New York.

CHAPTER 1: IN UTERO

14. Ezkurdia, I., et al., 'Multiple evidence strands suggest that there may be as few as 19,000 human protein-coding genes'. *Hum Mol Genet*, 2014. **23**(22): pp. 5866–78.

15. Darlington, C.L., *The Female Brain*. 2nd ed. Conceptual advances in brain research. 2009, Boca Raton, FL.: Taylor & Francis Group.

16. Vaitukaitis, J.L., 'Development of the home pregnancy test'. *Ann N Y Acad Sci*, 2004. **1038**: pp. 220–2.

17. Bale, T.L., 'The placenta and neurodevelopment: sex differences in prenatal vulnerability'. *Dialogues Clin Neurosci*, 2016. 18(4): pp. 459–64.

18. Blom, H.J., et al., 'Neural tube defects and folate: case far from closed'. *Nat Rev Neurosci*, 2006. **7**(9): pp. 724–31.

19. Wilhelm, D., S. Palmer and P. Koopman, 'Sex determination and gonadal development in mammals'. *Physiol Rev*, 2007. **87**(1): pp. 1–28.

20. Graves, J., 'Differences between men and women are more than the sum of their genes'. 2015, The Conversation.

21. De Mees, C., et al., 'Alpha-fetoprotein controls female fertility and prenatal development of the gonadotropin-releasing hormone pathway through an antiestrogenic action'. *Mol Cell Biol*, 2006. **26**(5): pp. 2012–18.

22. Fine, C., et al., 'Plasticity, plasticity, plasticity … and the rigid problem of sex'. *Trends Cogn Sci*, 2013. **17**(11): pp. 550–1.

23. Sacks, O., *The Man Who Mistook His Wife for a Hat*. 1985, London: Picador Classic.

24. Eriksson, P.S., et al., 'Neurogenesis in the adult human hippocampus'. *Nat Med*, 1998. **4**(11): pp. 1313–17.

25. Dennis, C.V., et al., 'Human adult neurogenesis across the ages: An immunohistochemical study'. *Neuropathol Appl Neurobiol*, 2016. **42**(7): pp. 621–38.

26. Wu, J., et al., 'Available Evidence of Association between Zika Virus and Microcephaly'. *Chin Med J (Engl)*, 2016. **129**(19): pp. 2347–56.

27. Wu, K.Y., et al., 'Vertical transmission of Zika virus targeting the radial glial cells affects cortex development of offspring mice'. *Cell Res*, 2016. **26**(6): pp. 645–54.

28. Ekblad, M., J. Korkeila and L. Lehtonen, 'Smoking during pregnancy affects foetal brain development'. *Acta Paediatr*, 2015. **104**(1): pp. 12–18.

29. Ramsay, H., et al., 'Smoking in pregnancy, adolescent mental health and cognitive performance in young adult offspring: results from a matched sample within a Finnish cohort'. *BMC Psychiatry*, 2016. **16**(1): p. 430.

30. Turner-Cobb, J.M., *Child Health Psychology: A biopsychosocial perspective*. 2014, Los Angeles: Sage.

31. DiPietro, J.A., et al., 'Maternal psychological distress during pregnancy in relation to child development at age two'. *Child Dev*, 2006. **77**(3): pp. 573–87.

32. King, S., et al., 'Using natural disasters to study the effects of prenatal maternal stress on child health and development'. *Birth Defects Res C Embryo Today*, 2012. **96**(4): pp. 273–88.

CHAPTER 2: CHILDHOOD

33. Jernigan, T.L., et al., 'Postnatal brain development: structural imaging of dynamic neurodevelopmental processes'. *Prog Brain Res*, 2011. **189**: pp. 77–92.

34. Lebel, C. and C. Beaulieu, 'Longitudinal development of human brain wiring continues from childhood into adulthood'. *J Neurosci*, 2011. **31**(30): pp. 10937–47.

35. Stiles, J. and T.L. Jernigan, 'The basics of brain development'. *Neuropsychol Rev*, 2010. **20**(4): pp. 327–48.

36. Newby, J., 'The New Science of Wisdom', in *Catalyst*. L. Heywood, Editor. 2006: ABC.

37. Gopnik, A., 'How babies think'. *Scientific American*, 2010 (July).

38. Takesian, A.E. and T.K. Hensch, 'Balancing plasticity/stablity across brain development', in *Progress in Brain Research*. 2013, Elsevier.

39. Fagiolini, M., et al., 'Specific GABAAA circuits for visual cortical plasticity'. *Science*, 2004. **303**(5664): pp. 1681–3.

40. Hensch, T.K., 'The Power of the Infant Brain'. *Sci Am*, 2016. **314**(2): pp. 64–9.

41. Friedmann, N. and D. Rusou, 'Critical period for first language: the crucial role of language input during the first year of life'. *Curr Opin Neurobiol*, 2015. **35**: pp. 27–34.

42. Kuhl, P.K. and A.R. Damasio, 'Language', in *Principles of Neural Science*, E.R. Kandel, J.H. Schwartz, T.M. Jessell, S.A. Siegelbaum, A.J. Hudspeth, Editors. 2013, New York: McGraw Hill Medical.

43. Preisler, G., 'Development of communication in children with sensory functional disabilities', in *The Wiley-Blackwell Handbook of Infant Development*. 2010, Wiley Blackwell: Chichester.

44. Sonuga-Barke, E.J., et al., 'Child-to-adult neurodevelopmental and mental health trajectories after early life deprivation: the young adult follow-up of the longitudinal English and Romanian Adoptees study'. *Lancet*, 2017.

45. Center on the Developing Child. 'Toxic Stress'. 2017 [cited 23 March 2017]; Available from: http://developingchild.harvard.edu/science/key-concepts/toxic-stress/.

46. Caspi, A., et al., 'Childhood forecasting of a small segment of the population with large economic burden'. *Nature Human Behaviour* 2016. **1**.

47. Liberty, K., et al., 'Behavior Problems and Post-traumatic Stress Symptoms in Children Beginning School: A Comparison of Pre- and Post-Earthquake Groups. '. *PLOS Currents Disasters.*, 2016. **1**.

48. Lupien, S.J., et al., 'Effects of stress throughout the lifespan on the brain, behaviour and cognition'. *Nat Rev Neurosci*, 2009. **10**(6): pp. 434–45.

49. Krugers, H.J., et al., 'Early life adversity: Lasting consequences for emotional learning'. *Neurobiol Stress*, 2017. **6**: pp. 14–21.

50. Heetkamp, T. and I. deTerte, 'PTSD and Resilience in Adolescents after New Zealand Earthquakes'. *New Zealand Journal of Psychology*, 2015. **44**(1).

51. Lambert, S., et al., 'Indigenous resilience through urban disaster: The Maori response to the 2010 and 2011 Christchurch Otautahi earthquakes'. *Proceedings of the International Indigenous Development Research Conference*, 2012. Auckland Ngä Pae o te Märamatanga.

52. Pasterski, V., S. Golombok and M. Hines, 'Sex differences in social behaviour', in *The Wiley Blackwell Handbook of Childhood Social Development*, P.K. Smith and C.H. Hart, Editors. 2014, Wiley Blackwell: Chichester.

53. Hines, M., et al., 'Prenatal androgen exposure alters girls' responses to information indicating gender-appropriate behaviour'. *Philos Trans R Soc Lond B Biol Sci*, 2016. **371**(1688): p. 20150125.

54. Kuiri-Hanninen, T., U. Sankilampi and L. Dunkel, 'Activation of the hypothalamic-pituitary-gonadal axis in infancy: minipuberty'. *Horm Res Paediatr*, 2014. **82**(2): pp. 73–80.

55. Lonsdorf, E.V., 'Sex differences in nonhuman primate behavioral development'. *J Neurosci Res*, 2017. **95**(1–2): pp. 213–21.

56. Robles de Medina, P.G., et al., 'Fetal behaviour does not differ between boys and girls'. *Early Hum Dev*, 2003. **73**(1–2): pp. 17–26.

57. Aznar, A. and H.R. Tenenbaum, 'Gender and age differences in parent-child emotion talk'. *Br J Dev Psychol*, 2015. **33**(1): pp. 148–55.

58.   Tenenbaum, H.R., S. Ford and B. Alkhedairy, 'Telling stories: gender differences in peers' emotion talk and communication style'. *Br J Dev Psychol*, 2011. **29**(Pt 4): pp. 707–21.

59.   Leman, P.J. and H.R. Tenenbaum, 'Practising gender: children's relationships and the development of gendered behaviour and beliefs'. *Br J Dev Psychol*, 2011. **29**(Pt 2): pp. 153–7.

60.   Maney, D.L., 'Just like a circus: the public consumption of sex differences'. *Curr Top Behav Neurosci*, 2015. **19**: pp. 279–96.

61.   von Stumm, S., T. Chamorro-Premuzic and A. Furnham, 'Decomposing self-estimates of intelligence: structure and sex differences across 12 nations'. *Br J Psychol*, 2009. **100**(Pt 2): pp. 429–42.

62.   Bian, L., S. J. Leslie and A. Cimpian, 'Gender stereotypes about intellectual ability emerge early and influence children's interests'. *Science*, 2017. **355**(6323): pp. 389–391.

63.   Goodwin, K., *Raising your child in a digital world*. 2016, Sydney: Finch Publishing.

CHAPTER 3: PUBERTY

64.   Oberfield, S.E., A.B. Sopher and A.T. Gerken, 'Approach to the girl with early onset of pubic hair'. *J Clin Endocrinol Metab*, 2011. **96**(6): pp. 1610–22.

65.   Mundy, L.K., et al., 'Adrenarche and the Emotional and Behavioral Problems of Late Childhood'. *J Adolesc Health*, 2015. **57**(6): pp. 608–16.

66.   Delany, F.M., et al., 'Depression, immune function, and early adrenarche in children'. *Psychoneuroendocrinology*, 2016. **63**: pp. 228–34.

67.   Whittle, S., et al., 'Associations between early adrenarche, affective brain function and mental health in children'. *Soc Cogn Affect Neurosci*, 2015. **10**(9): pp. 1282–90.

68.   Klauser, P., et al., 'Reduced frontal white matter volume in children with early onset of adrenarche'. *Psychoneuroendocrinology*, 2015. **52**: pp. 111–18.

69.   Byrne, M.L., et al., 'A systematic review of adrenarche as a sensitive period in neurobiological development and mental health'. *Dev Cogn Neurosci*, 2017. **25**: pp. 12–28.

70.   Australian Institute of Family Studies, 'The Longitudinal Study of Australian Children Annual Statistical Report 2015'. 2016, Commonwealth of Australia: Melbourne.

71.   Seminara, S.B. and W.F. Crowley, Jr., 'Kisspeptin and GPR54: discovery of a novel pathway in reproduction'. *J Neuroendocrinol*, 2008. **20**(6): pp. 727–31.

72. de Roux, N., et al., 'Hypogonadotropic hypogonadism due to loss of function of the KiSS1–derived peptide receptor GPR54'. *Proc Natl Acad Sci U S A*, 2003. **100**(19): pp. 10972–6.

73. Herman-Giddens, M.E., et al., 'Secondary sexual characteristics and menses in young girls seen in office practice: a study from the Pediatric Research in Office Settings network'. *Pediatrics*, 1997. **99**(4): pp. 505–12.

74. Biro, F.M., et al., 'Onset of breast development in a longitudinal cohort'. *Pediatrics*, 2013. **132**(6): pp. 1019–27.

75. Greenspan, L. and J. Deardorff, *The New Puberty. How to navigate early development in today's girls.* 2014, New York: Rodale.

76. Aksglaede, L., et al., 'Age at puberty and the emerging obesity epidemic'. *PLoS One*, 2009. **4**(12): p. e8450.

77. Balzer, B.W., et al., 'The effects of estradiol on mood and behavior in human female adolescents: a systematic review'. *Eur J Pediatr*, 2015. **174**(3): pp. 289–98.

CHAPTER 4: THE MENSTRUAL CYCLE

78. Rosewarne, L., *Periods in Pop Culture: Menstruation in Film and Television* 2012, London: Lexington Books.

79. Angier, N., *Woman. An Intimate Geography.* 2014, London: Virago.

80. Toffoletto, S., et al., 'Emotional and cognitive functional imaging of estrogen and progesterone effects in the female human brain: a systematic review'. *Psychoneuroendocrinology*, 2014. **50**: pp. 28–52.

81. Sundström-Poromaa, I. and M. Gingnell, 'Menstrual cycle influence on cognitive function and emotion processing – from a reproductive perspective'. *Front Neurosci*, 2014. **8**: p. 380.

82. Ferree, N.K., R. Kamat and L. Cahill, 'Influences of menstrual cycle position and sex hormone levels on spontaneous intrusive recollections following emotional stimuli'. *Conscious Cogn*, 2011. **20**(4): pp. 1154–62.

83. McCarthy, M.M., 'Multifaceted origins of sex differences in the brain'. *Philos Trans R Soc Lond B Biol Sci*, 2016. **371**(1688): p. 20150106.

84. Bramble, M.S., et al., 'Effects of chromosomal sex and hormonal influences on shaping sex differences in brain and behavior: Lessons from cases of disorders of sex development'. *J Neurosci Res*, 2017. **95**(1–2): pp. 65–74.

85. Irwing, P. and R. Lynn, 'Sex differences in means and variability on the progressive matrices in university students: a meta-analysis'. *Br J Psychol*, 2005. **96**(Pt 4): pp. 505–24.

86. Blinkhorn, S., 'Intelligence: a gender bender'. *Nature*, 2005. **438**(7064): pp. 31–2.

87. Direkvand-Moghadam, A., et al., 'Epidemiology of Premenstrual Syndrome (PMS)-A Systematic Review and Meta-Analysis Study'. *J Clin Diagn Res*, 2014. **8**(2): pp. 106–9.

88. Romans, S., et al., 'Mood and the menstrual cycle: a review of prospective data studies'. *Gend Med*, 2012. **9**(5): pp. 361–84.

89. Romans, S.E., et al., 'Mood and the menstrual cycle'. *Psychother Psychosom*, 2013. **82**(1): pp. 53–60.

90. Ussher, J., 'The myth of premenstrual moodiness', in The Conversation. 2012.

91. Kulkarni, J., 'PMS is real and denying its existence harms women', in The Conversation. 2012.

92. Gehlert, S., et al., 'The prevalence of premenstrual dysphoric disorder in a randomly selected group of urban and rural women'. *Psychol Med*, 2009. **39**(1): pp. 129–36.

93. Comasco, E. and I. Sundström-Poromaa, 'Neuroimaging the Menstrual Cycle and Premenstrual Dysphoric Disorder'. *Curr Psychiatry Rep*, 2015. **17**(10): p. 77.

94. Romans, S.E., et al., 'Crying, oral contraceptive use and the menstrual cycle'. *J Affect Disord*, 2017. **208**: pp. 272–7.

95. Skovlund, C.W., et al., 'Association of Hormonal Contraception With Depression'. *JAMA Psychiatry*, 2016. **73**(11): pp. 1154–62.

96. Wise, J., 'Hormonal contraception use among teenagers linked to depression'. *BMJ*, 2016. **354**: p. i5289.

97. Zethraeus, N., et al., 'A first-choice combined oral contraceptive influences general well-being in healthy women: a double-blind, randomized, placebo-controlled trial'. *Fertil Steril*, 2017. **107**(5): pp. 1238–45.

98. Iversen, L., et al., 'Lifetime cancer risk and combined oral contraceptives: the Royal College of General Practitioners' Oral Contraception Study'. *Am J Obstet Gynecol*, 2017.

99. Pletzer, B.A. and H.H. Kerschbaum, '50 years of hormonal contraception – time to find out, what it does to our brain'. *Front Neurosci*, 2014. **8**: p. 256.

CHAPTER 5: THE TEENAGE BRAIN

100. Choudhury, S., K.A. McKinney and M. Merten, 'Rebelling against the brain: public engagement with the "neurological adolescent"'. *Soc Sci Med*, 2012. **74**(4): pp. 565–73.

101. Walhovd, K.B., et al., 'Through Thick and Thin: a Need to Reconcile Contradictory Results on Trajectories in Human Cortical Development'. *Cereb Cortex*, 2017. **27**(2): pp. 1472–81.

102. Giedd, J.N., 'The amazing teen brain'. *Scientific American*, 2015 (June).

103. Peper, J.S., et al., 'Sex steroids and brain structure in pubertal boys and girls: a mini-review of neuroimaging studies'. *Neuroscience*, 2011. **191**: pp. 28–37.

104. Ladouceur, C.D., et al., 'White matter development in adolescence: the influence of puberty and implications for affective disorders'. *Dev Cogn Neurosci*, 2012. **2**(1): pp. 36–54.

105. Damour, L., *Untangled: Guiding Teenage Girls through the Seven Transitions into Adulthood*. 2016, New York: Penguin Random House.

106. Cooke. K., *Girl Stuff. A full-on guide to the teen years*. 2013, Australia: Penguin Random House.

107. Purdue University, 'Pain of ostracism can be deep, long-lasting'. 2011, ScienceDaily, 6 June 2011.

108. Sebastian, C.L., et al., 'Developmental influences on the neural bases of responses to social rejection: implications of social neuroscience for education'. *Neuroimage*, 2011. **57**(3): pp. 686–94.

109. Berns, G.S., et al., 'Neural mechanisms of the influence of popularity on adolescent ratings of music'. *Neuroimage*, 2010. **49**(3): pp. 2687–96.

110. Eisenberger, N.I., 'The pain of social disconnection: examining the shared neural underpinnings of physical and social pain'. *Nat Rev Neurosci*, 2012. **13**(6): pp. 421–34.

111. Dewall, C.N., et al., 'Acetaminophen reduces social pain: behavioral and neural evidence'. *Psychol Sci*, 2010. **21**(7): pp. 931–7.

112. Stephanou, K., et al., 'Hard to look on the bright side: Neural correlates of impaired emotion regulation in depressed youth'. *Soc Cogn Affect Neurosci*, 2017.

113. Guyer, A.E., J.S. Silk and E.E. Nelson, 'The neurobiology of the emotional adolescent: From the inside out'. *Neurosci Biobehav Rev*, 2016. **70**: pp. 74–85.

114. Poulton, R., T.E. Moffitt and P.A. Silva, 'The Dunedin Multidisciplinary Health and Development Study: overview of the first 40 years, with an eye to the future'. *Soc Psychiatry Psychiatr Epidemiol*, 2015. **50**(5): pp. 679–93.

115. Nelson, J.A., 'The power of stereotyping and confirmation bias to overwhelm accurate assessment: the case of economics, gender, and risk aversion'. *Journal of Economic Methodology*, 2014. 21(3): pp. 211–31.

116. Fine, C., *Testosterone Rex: Unmaking the Myths of Our Gendered Minds*. 2017, Sydney: Icon Boks.

117. Somerville, L.H., 'Special issue on the teenage brain: Sensitivity to social evaluation'. *Curr Dir Psychol Sci*, 2013. **22**(2): pp. 121–7.

118. Gardner, M. and L. Steinberg, 'Peer influence on risk taking, risk preference, and risky decision making in adolescence and adulthood: an experimental study'. *Dev Psychol*, 2005. **41**(4): pp. 625–35.

119. Blakemore, S.J., 'Adolescent brain development', M. Costandi, Editor. 2014, The Wellcome Trust.

CHAPTER 6: DEPRESSION AND ANXIETY

120. Lewinsohn, P.M., et al., 'Separation anxiety disorder in childhood as a risk factor for future mental illness'. *J Am Acad Child Adolesc Psychiatry*, 2008. **47**(5): pp. 548–55.

121. North, B., M. Gross and S. Smith, 'Study confirms HSC exams source of major stress to adolescents'. 2015, The Conversation.

122. Kuehner, C., 'Why is depression more common among women than among men?'. *Lancet Psychiatry*, 2016. **4**(2): pp. 146–58.

123. Solomon, A., 'Depression: the secret we share'. 2013, TED Talk.

124. *beyondblue*. '*beyondblue: the facts*'. 2017 [cited 2017; Available from: https://www.beyondblue.org.au/the-facts].

125. Craske, M.G., et al., 'Anxiety disorders'. *Nat Rev Dis Primers*, 2017. **3**: p. 17024.

126. *beyondblue*, 'Types of Anxiety: PTSD'. 2017.

127. Schaefer, J.D., et al., 'Enduring mental health: Prevalence and prediction'. *J Abnorm Psychol*, 2017. **126**(2): pp. 212–24.

128. *beyondblue*. '*Youth beyondblue: stats and facts*'. 2017; Available from: https://www.youthbeyondblue.com/footer/stats-and-facts.

129. Schmaal, L., et al., 'Subcortical brain alterations in major depressive disorder: findings from the ENIGMA Major Depressive Disorder working group'. *Mol Psychiatry*, 2016. **21**(6): pp. 806–12.

130. Anthes, E., 'Depression: A change of mind'. *Nature*, 2014. **515**(7526): pp. 185–7.

131. Jorm, A.F., et al., 'A guide to what works for depression'. 2013, *beyondblue*: Melbourne.

132. Gressier, F., R. Calati and A. Serretti, '5–HTTLPR and gender differences in affective disorders: A systematic review'. *J Affect Disord*, 2016. **190**: pp. 193–207.

133. Caspi, A., et al., 'Moderation of the effect of adolescent-onset cannabis use on adult psychosis by a functional polymorphism in the catechol-O-methyltransferase gene: longitudinal evidence of a gene x environment interaction'. *Biol Psychiatry*, 2005. **57**(10): pp. 1117–27.

134. Belsky, J. and M. Pluess, 'Beyond diathesis stress: differential susceptibility to environmental influences'. *Psychol Bull*, 2009. **135**(6): pp. 885–908.

135. Caspi, A., et al., 'Genetic sensitivity to the environment: the case of the serotonin transporter gene and its implications for studying complex diseases and traits'. *Am J Psychiatry*, 2010. **167**(5): pp. 509–27.

136. Culverhouse, R.C., et al., 'Collaborative meta-analysis finds no evidence of a strong interaction between stress and 5–HTTLPR genotype contributing to the development of depression'. *Mol Psychiatry*, 2017.

137. Riecher-Rossler, A., 'Sex and gender differences in mental disorders'. *Lancet Psychiatry*, 2017. **4**(1): pp. 8–9.

138. Kulkarni, J., 'Hormones actually a great protector of women's health'. 2011, The Conversation.

139. Li, S.H. and B.M. Graham, 'Why are women so vulnerable to anxiety, trauma-related and stress-related disorders? The potential role of sex hormones'. *Lancet Psychiatry*, 2017. **4**(1): pp. 73–82.

140. Merz, C.J. and O.T. Wolf, 'Sex differences in stress effects on emotional learning'. *J Neurosci Res*, 2017. **95**(1–2): pp. 93–105.

141. Bryant, R.A., et al., 'The association between menstrual cycle and traumatic memories'. *J Affect Disord*, 2011. **131**(1–3): pp. 398–401.

142. Ferree, N. K., M. Wheeler and L. Cahill, 'The influence of emergency contraception on post-traumatic stress symptoms following sexual assault'. *J Forensic Nurs*, 2012. **8**(3): pp. 122–30.

143. Mordecai, K.L., et al., 'Cortisol reactivity and emotional memory after psychosocial stress in oral contraceptive users'. *J Neurosci Res*, 2017. **95**(1–2): pp. 126–35.

144. Oldehinkel, A. J. & E.M. Bouma, 'Sensitivity to the depressogenic effect of stress and HPA-axis reactivity in adolescence: a review of gender differences'. *Neurosci Biobehav*, 2011. **35**(8): pp. 1757–70.

145. Dantzer, R. and K.W. Kelley, 'Twenty years of research on cytokine-induced sickness behavior'. *Brain Behav Immun*, 2007. **21**(2): pp. 153–60.

146. Raison, C.L., et al., 'A randomized controlled trial of the tumor necrosis factor antagonist infliximab for treatment-resistant depression: the role of baseline inflammatory biomarkers'. *JAMA Psychiatry*, 2013. **70**(1): pp. 31–41.

147. Pariante, C. M., 'Why are depressed patients inflamed? A reflection on 20 years of research on depression, glucocorticoid resistance and inflammation'. *Eur Neuropsychopharmacol*, 2017. **27**(6): pp. 554–9.

148. World Health Organization and London School of Hygiene and Tropical Medicine, 'Preventing intimate partner and sexual violence against women. Taking action and generating evidence'. 2010.

149. Chen, Y.Y., et al., 'Women's status and depressive symptoms: a multilevel analysis'. *Soc Sci Med*, 2005. **60**(1): pp. 49–60.

150. Van de Velde, S., et al., 'Macro-level gender equality and depression in men and women in Europe'. *Sociol Health Illn*, 2013. **35**(5): pp. 682–98.

CHAPTER 7: SEX, LOVE AND NEUROBIOLOGY

151. Suleiman, A.B., et al., 'Becoming a sexual being: The "elephant in the room" of adolescent brain development'. *Dev Cogn Neurosci*, 2017. **25**: pp. 209–20.

152. Wedekind, C., et al., 'MHC-dependent mate preferences in humans'. *Proc Biol Sci*, 1995. **260**(1359): pp. 245–9.

153. Ober, C., 'HLA and fertility'. *Am J Hum Genet*, 1995. **57**(5): pp. 1242–3.

154. Durante, K.M., et al., 'Ovulation leads women to perceive sexy cads as good dads'. *J Pers Soc Psychol*, 2012. **103**(2): pp. 292–305.

155. Brooks, R., 'Round 2: Ovulatory Cycles and Shifting Preferences'. 2014, The Conversation.

156. Roney, J.R. and Z.L. Simmons, 'Hormonal predictors of sexual motivation in natural menstrual cycles'. *Horm Behav*, 2013. **63**(4): pp. 636–45.

157. Dennerstein, L., et al., 'Hormones, mood, sexuality, and the menopausal transition'. *Fertil Steril*, 2002. **77 Suppl 4**: pp. S42–8.

158. Pastor, Z., K. Holla, and R. Chmel, 'The influence of combined oral contraceptives on female sexual desire: a systematic review'. *Eur J Contracept Reprod Health Care*, 2013. **18**(1): pp. 27–43.

159. Meston, C.M. and D.M. Buss, 'Why humans have sex'. *Arch Sex Behav*, 2007. **36**(4): pp. 477–507.

160. Whipple, B. and K. Brash-McGreer, 'Management of female sexual dysfunction', in *Sexual function in people with disability and chronic illness: a health professional's guide*, M.L. Sipski and C.J. Alexander, Editors. 1997, Gaithersburg: Aspen.

161. 'What you need to know. Female Sexual Response.', in http://www.arhp.org/Publications-and-Resources, A.o.R.H. Professionals. Editor. 2008.

162. Basson, R., 'Female sexual response: the role of drugs in the management of sexual dysfunction'. *Obstet Gynecol*, 2001. **98**(2): pp. 350–3.

163. Nagoski, E., *Come as You Are: the surprising new science that will transform your sex life*. 2015, New York: Simon & Schuster.

164. Georgiadis, J.R., M.L. Kringelbach and J.G. Pfaus, 'Sex for fun: a synthesis of human and animal neurobiology'. *Nat Rev Urol*, 2012. **9**(9): pp. 486–98.

165. Goldstein, I., et al., 'Hypoactive Sexual Desire Disorder: International Society for the Study of Women's Sexual Health (ISSWSH) Expert Consensus Panel Review'. *Mayo Clin Proc*, 2017. **92**(1): pp. 114–128.

166. Kingsberg, S.A., A.H. Clayton, and J.G. Pfaus, 'The Female Sexual Response: Current Models, Neurobiological Underpinnings and Agents Currently Approved or Under Investigation for the Treatment of Hypoactive Sexual Desire Disorder'. *CNS Drugs*, 2015. **29**(11): pp. 915–33.

167. Lucke, J., 'Weekly Dose: flibanserin, the drug that gives women one extra sexually satisfying experience every two months'. 2016: The Conversation.

168. 'Female Sex Drive', in *Catalyst*, D.J. Newby, Editor. 2015, ABC.

169. Basson, R., 'Testosterone therapy for reduced libido in women'. *Ther Adv Endocrinol Metab*, 2010. **1**(4): pp. 155–64.

170. University of Melbourne, 'Menopause dashes sex life'. 2002, Melbourne: Eureka Alert.

171. Bergner, D., *What Do Women Want?: Adventures in the Science of Female Desire*. 2014, New York: HarperCollins.

172. Perel, E., *Mating in Captivity: Sex, Lies and Domestic Bliss*. 2007, London: Hodder & Stoughton

173. Dickson, N., et al., 'Stability and change in same-sex attraction, experience, and identity by sex and age in a New Zealand birth cohort'. *Arch Sex Behav*, 2013. **42**(5): pp. 753–63.

174. Chantry, K. 'The transgender bathroom contoversy: four essential reads'. 2017 [cited 2017 March 4th]; Available from: https://theconversation.com/the-transgender-bathroom-controversy-four-essential-reads-72635.

175. Fusion. 'Massive Millennial Poll'. 2015; Available from: http://fusion.net/story/42216/half-of-young-people-believe-gender-isnt-limited-to-male-and-female/.

176. Zeki, S. and J.P. Romaya, 'The brain reaction to viewing faces of opposite- and same-sex romantic partners'. *PLoS One*, 2010. **5**(12): p. e15802.

177. Meston, C.M., R.J. Levin, M.L. Sipski, E.M. Hull and J.R. Heiman, 'Women's Orgasm'. *Annu Rev Sex Res*, 2004. **15**(1): pp. 173–257.

178. O'Connell, H.E., K.V. Sanjeevan, and J.M. Hutson, 'Anatomy of the clitoris'. *J Urol*, 2005. **174**(4 Pt 1): pp. 1189–95.

179. Sample, I., 'Female orgasm captured in series of brain scans', in *The Guardian*. 2011.

180. Kontula, O. and A. Miettinen, 'Determinants of female sexual orgasms'. *Socioaffect Neurosci Psychol*, 2016. **6**: p. 31624.

181. Coria-Avila, G.A., et al., 'The role of orgasm in the development and shaping of partner preferences'. *Socioaffect Neurosci Psychol*, 2016. **6**: p. 31815.

182. King, R., M. Dempsey and K.A. Valentine, 'Measuring sperm backflow following female orgasm: a new method'. *Socioaffect Neurosci Psychol*, 2016. **6**: p. 31927.

183. Earp, B.D., et al., 'Addicted to love: What is love addiction and when should it be treated?'. *Philos Psychiatr Psychol*, 2017. **24**(1): pp. 77–92.

184. Fisher, H.E., et al., 'Intense, Passionate, Romantic Love: A Natural Addiction? How the Fields That Investigate Romance and Substance Abuse Can Inform Each Other'. *Front Psychol*, 2016. **7**: p. 687.

185. Acevedo, B.P., et al., 'Neural correlates of long-term intense romantic love'. *Soc Cogn Affect Neurosci*, 2012. **7**(2): pp. 145–59.

186. Carter, C.S. and S.W. Porges, 'The biochemistry of love: an oxytocin hypothesis'. *EMBO reports*, 2013. **14**(1).

187. Pedersen, C.A. and A.J. Prange, Jr., 'Induction of maternal behavior in virgin rats after intracerebroventricular administration of oxytocin'. *Proc Natl Acad Sci U S A*, 1979. **76**(12): pp. 6661–5.

188. Churchland, P.S. and P. Winkielman, 'Modulating social behavior with oxytocin: how does it work? What does it mean?'. *Horm Behav*, 2012. **61**(3): pp. 392–9.

189. Patoine, B., 'One Molecule for Love, Trust, and Morality? Separating Hype from Hope in the Oxytocin Research Explosion'. 2013: The Dana Foundation.

190. McGonigal, K., 'How to make stress your friend'. 2013, TED Talk.

191. Kosfeld, M., et al., 'Oxytocin increases trust in humans'. *Nature*, 2005. **435**(7042): pp. 673–6.

192. Damasio, A., 'Brain Trust'. *Nature*, 2005. **435**(2 June): pp. 571–2.

193.   Kemp, A.H. and A. Gustella, 'The dark side of the love drug –
        oxytocin linked to gloating, envy and aggression'. 2011: The
        Conversation.

194.   Shen, H., 'Neuroscience: The hard science of oxytocin'. *Nature*, 2015.
        522(7557): pp. 410–12.

CHAPTER 8: PREGNANCY AND MOTHERHOOD

195.   Hoekzema, E., et al., 'Pregnancy leads to long-lasting changes in
        human brain structure'. *Nat Neurosci*, 2017. **20**(2): pp. 287–96.

196.   Pereira, M. and A. Ferreira, 'Neuroanatomical and neurochemical basis
        of parenting: Dynamic coordination of motivational, affective and
        cognitive processes'. *Hormones and Behavior*, 2016. (77): pp. 72–85.

197.   Levy, F., G. Gheusi and M. Keller, 'Plasticity of the parental brain: a
        case for neurogenesis'. *J Neuroendocrinol*, 2011. **23**(11): pp. 984–93.

198.   Hrdy, S.B., 'Variable postpartum responsiveness among humans
        and other primates with "cooperative breeding": A comparative and
        evolutionary perspective'. *Horm Behav*, 2016. **77**: pp. 272–83.

199.   Brunton, P.J. and J.A. Russell, 'The expectant brain: adapting for
        motherhood'. *Nat Rev Neurosci*, 2008. **9**(1): pp. 11–25.

200.   Russell, J.A., A.J. Douglas and C.D. Ingram, 'Brain preparations
        for maternity – adaptive changes in behavioral and neuroendocrine
        systems during pregnancy and lactation. An overview'. *Prog Brain Res*,
        2001. **133**: pp. 1–38.

201.   Grattan, D.R. and I.C. Kokay, 'Prolactin: a pleiotropic neuroendocrine
        hormone'. *J Neuroendocrinol*, 2008. **20**(6): pp. 752–63.

202.   Grattan, D.R., '60 years of neuroendocrinology: The hypothalamo-
        prolactin axis'. *J Endocrinol*, 2015. **226**(2): pp. T101–22.

203.   NICE, 'NICE public health guidance 27: Weight management before,
        during and after pregnancy'. 2010, National Institute for Health and
        Clinical Excellence: London.

204.   Committee to Reexamine Institute of Medicine Pregnancy Weight
        Guidelines, 'Weight gain during pregnancy: reexamining the
        guidelines'. 2009, National Academies Press, Washington DC.

205.   de Jersey, S.J., et al., 'A prospective study of pregnancy weight gain in
        Australian women'. *Aust NZ J Obstet Gynaecol*, 2012. **52**(6): pp. 545–51.

206.   Torner, L., et al., 'Anxiolytic and anti-stress effects of brain prolactin:
        improved efficacy of antisense targeting of the prolactin receptor by
        molecular modeling'. *J Neurosci*, 2001. **21**(9): pp. 3207–14.

207. Gustafson, P., S.J. Bunn and D.R. Grattan, 'The role of prolactin in the suppression of Crh mRNA expression during pregnancy and lactation in the mouse'. *J Neuroendocrinol*, 2017. **29**(9).

208. Buckwalter, J.G., D.K. Buckwalter, B.W. Bluestein and F.Z. Stanczyk, 'Pregnancy and postpartum: changes in cognition and mood', in *The Maternal Brain. Progress in Brain Research*. 2001, Elsevier.

209. Logan, D.M., K.R. Hill et al., 'How do memory and attention change with pregnancy and childbirth? A controlled longitudinal examination of neuropsychological functioning in pregnant and postpartum women'. *Clin Exp Neuropsychol*. **36**(5): pp.528–39.

210. Christensen, H., C. Poyser, P. Pollitt and J. Cubis, 'Pregnancy may confer a selective cognitive advantage'. *Journal of Reproductive and Infant Psychology*, 1999. **17**(1): pp. 7–25.

211. Casey, P., 'A longitudinal study of cognitive performance during pregnancy and new motherhood'. *Archives of Women's Mental Health*, 2000. **3**(2): pp. 65–76.

212. Ellison, K., *The Mommy Brain: How Motherhood Makes Us Smarter*. 2005, New York: Basic Books.

213. Stern D.N. and N. Bruschweiler-Stern, *The Birth Of A Mother: How The Motherhood Experience Changes You Forever*. 1998, New York: Basic Books.

214. Kim, P., L. Strathearn and J.E. Swain, 'The maternal brain and its plasticity in humans'. *Horm Behav*, 2016. **77**: pp. 113–23.

215. Moore, E.R., et al., 'Early skin-to-skin contact for mothers and their healthy newborn infants'. *Cochrane Database Syst Rev*, 2016. **11**: p. CD003519.

216. Rosenblatt, J.S., 'Nonhormonal basis of maternal behavior in the rat'. *Science* 1967. **156**(3781): pp. 1512–14.

217. Lingle, S. and T. Riede, 'Deer Mothers are Sensitive to Infant Distress Vocalizations of Diverse Mammalian Species'. *The American Naturalist*, 2014. **184**(4): pp. 510–522.

218. Feldman, R., 'The neurobiology of mammalian parenting and the biosocial context of human caregiving'. *Horm Behav*, 2016. **77**: pp. 3–17.

219. Gordon, I., et al., 'Testosterone, oxytocin, and the development of human parental care'. *Horm Behav*, 2017. **93**: pp. 184–192.

220. Krol, K.M., et al., 'Breastfeeding experience differentially impacts recognition of happiness and anger in mothers'. *Sci Rep*, 2014. **4**: p. 7006.

221. Hahn-Holbrook, J., et al, 'Maternal defense: breast feeding increases aggression by reducing stress'. *Psychol Sci*, 2011. 22(10): pp. 1288–1295.

222. Donato, J., Jr. and R. Frazao, 'Interactions between prolactin and kisspeptin to control reproduction'. *Arch Endocrinol Metab*, 2016. **60**(6): pp. 587–95.

223. Patton, C.C., 'Prediction of perinatal depression from adolescence and before conception (VIHCS): 20-year prospective cohort study'. *Lancet*, 2015. 386(9996): pp. 875–883.

224. Loxton, D. and J. Lucke, 'Reproductive health: Findings from the Australian Longitudinal Study on Women's Health'. 2009: Australian Government Department of Health.

225. Weaver, J.J. and J.M. Ussher, 'How motherhood changes life – a discourse analytic study with mothers of young children'. *Journal of Reproductive and Infant Psychology*, 2007. **15**(1): pp. 51–68.

CHAPTER 9: MENOPAUSE

226. Cooke, K., *Women's Stuff*. 2011, London: Penguin Random House.

227. Campbell, K.E., et al., 'The trajectory of negative mood and depressive symptoms over two decades'. *Maturitas*, 2017. **95**: pp. 36–41.

228. Brinton, R.D., et al., 'Perimenopause as a neurological transition state'. *Nat Rev Endocrinol*, 2015. **11**(7): pp. 393–405.

229. Brent, L.J., et al., 'Ecological knowledge, leadership, and the evolution of menopause in killer whales'. *Curr Biol*, 2015. **25**(6): pp. 746–50.

230. Rettberg, J.R., J. Yao and R.D. Brinton, 'Estrogen: a master regulator of bioenergetic systems in the brain and body'. *Front Neuroendocrinol*, 2014. **35**(1): pp. 8–30.

231. Freedman, R.R., 'Menopausal hot flashes: mechanisms, endocrinology, treatment'. *J Steroid Biochem Mol Biol*, 2014. **142**: pp. 115–20.

232. Hardy, J.D. and E.F. Du Bois, 'Differences between Men and Women in Their Response to Heat and Cold'. *Proc Natl Acad Sci USA*, 1940. **26**(6): pp. 389–98.

233. Charkoudian, N. and N.S. Stachenfeld, 'Reproductive hormone influences on thermoregulation in women'. *Compr Physiol*, 2014. **4**(2): pp. 793–804.

234. Prague, J.K., et al, 'Neurokinin 3 receptor antagonism as a novel treatment for menopausal hot flushes: a phase 2, randomised, double-blind, placebo-controlled trial'. *Lancet*, 2017. 389(10081): pp. 1809–1820.

235. Freedman, R.R., et al., 'Cortical activation during menopausal hot flashes'. *Fertil Steril*, 2006. **85**(3): pp. 674–8.

236. Berecki-Gisolf, J., N. Begum and A.J. Dobson, 'Symptoms reported by women in midlife: menopausal transition or aging?'. *Menopause*, 2009. **16**(5): pp. 1021–9.

237. Ciano, C., et al., 'Longitudinal Study of Insomnia Symptoms Among Women During Perimenopause'. *J Obstet Gynecol Neonatal Nurs*, 2017. **46**(6): pp. 804–13.

238. Grandner, M.A., 'Sleep, Health, and Society'. *Sleep Med Clin*, 2017. **12**(1): pp. 1–22.

239. Mong, J.A. and D.M. Cusmano, 'Sex differences in sleep: impact of biological sex and sex steroids'. *Philos Trans R Soc Lond B Biol Sci*, 2016. **371**(1688): p. 20150110.

240. Allmen, T., *Menopause Confidential. A Doctor Reveals the Secrets to Thriving Through Midlife.* 2016, New York: HarperCollins.

241. Gervais, N.J., J.A. Mong and A. Lacreuse, 'Ovarian hormones, sleep and cognition across the adult female lifespan: An integrated perspective'. *Front Neuroendocrinol*, 2017. **47**: pp. 134–53.

242. Adan, A. and V. Natale, 'Gender differences in morningness-eveningness preference'. *Chronobiol Int*, 2002. **19**(4): pp. 709–20.

243. Baker, F.C., et al., 'Insomnia in women approaching menopause: Beyond perception'. *Psychoneuroendocrinology*, 2015. **60**: pp. 96–104.

244. de Zambotti, M., et al., 'Magnitude of the impact of hot flashes on sleep in perimenopausal women'. *Fertil Steril*, 2014. **102**(6): pp. 1708–15 e1.

245. Kulkarni, J., 'There's no "rushing women's syndrome" but hormones affect mental health'. 2014, The Conversation.

246. Campbell, K.E., et al., 'Impact of menopausal status on negative mood and depressive symptoms in a longitudinal sample spanning 20 years'. *Menopause*, 2017. **24**(5): pp. 490–6.

247. Weber, M.T., P.M. Maki and M.P. McDermott, 'Cognition and mood in perimenopause: a systematic review and meta-analysis'. *J Steroid Biochem Mol Biol*, 2014. **142**: pp. 90–8.

248. Alzheimer's Australia. 'About demenita and memory loss'. Accessed 2017; Available from: https://www.fightdementia.org.au/about-dementia/memory-loss/memory-changes.

249. The Jean Hailes Foundation, 'Menopause Management'. 2017.

250. Pinkerton, J.V., 'Changing the conversation about hormone therapy'. *Menopause*, 2017. **24**(9): pp. 991–3.

251. The North American Menopause Society, 'The 2017 hormone therapy position statement of The North American Menopause Society'. *Menopause*, 2017. **24**(7): pp. 728–53.

252. Wilson, R.A. and T.A. Wilson, 'The Basic Philosophy of Estrogen Maintenance'. *The Journal of the American Geriatrics Society* 1972. **20**(11): pp. 521–523.

253. Hersh, A.L., M.L. Stefanick and R.S. Stafford, 'National use of postmenopausal hormone therapy: annual trends and response to recent evidence'. *JAMA*, 2004. **291**(1): pp. 47–53.

254. WHI. Available from: http://www.whi.org/.

255. Million Women Study; Available from: http://www.millionwomenstudy.org/.

256. Nurses' Health Study, Available from: http://www.nurseshealthstudy.org/.

257. 'Effects of estrogen or estrogen/progestin regimens on heart disease risk factors in postmenopausal women. The Postmenopausal Estrogen/Progestin Interventions (PEPI) Trial. The Writing Group for the PEPI Trial'. *JAMA*, 1995. **273**(3): pp. 199–208.

258. 'Study of Women's Health Across the Nation (SWAN)'. Available from: http://www.swanstudy.org/.

259. Shumaker, S.A., et al., 'Estrogen plus progestin and the incidence of dementia and mild cognitive impairment in postmenopausal women: the Women's Health Initiative Memory Study: a randomized controlled trial'. *JAMA*, 2003. **289**: pp. 2651–62.

260. Million Women Study, C., 'Breast cancer and hormone-replacement therapy in the Million Women Study'. *Lancet*, 2003. **362**(9382): pp. 419–27.

261. Cancer Council Australia. 'Breast Cancer'. 2017; Available from: http://www.cancer.org.au/about-cancer/types-of-cancer/breast-cancer/.

262. Barbieri, R.L., 'Patient education: Menopausal hormone therapy (Beyond the Basics)', K.A. Martin, Editor. 2017: UpToDate.

263. Cintron, D., et al., 'Efficacy of menopausal hormone therapy on sleep quality: systematic review and meta-analysis'. *Endocrine*, 2017. **55**(3): pp. 702–11.

264. Martin, K.A. and R.L. Barbieri, 'Treatment of menopausal symptoms with hormone therapy', in UpToDate, K.A. Martin, Editor. 2017.

265. Davison, S.L., et al., 'Testosterone improves verbal learning and memory in postmenopausal women: Results from a pilot study'. *Maturitas*, 2011. **70**(3): pp. 307–11.

266. Manson, J.E., et al., 'Menopausal Hormone Therapy and Long-term All-Cause and Cause-Specific Mortality: The Women's Health Initiative Randomized Trials'. *JAMA*, 2017. **318**(10): pp. 927–38.

267. MacLennan, A.H., V.W. Henderson, B.J. Paine, J. Mathias, E.N. Ramsay, P. Ryan, N.P. Stocks and A.W. Taylor, 'Hormone therapy, timing of initiation, and cognition in women aged older than 60 years: the REMEMBER pilot study'. *Menopause*, 2006. **13**: pp. 28–36.

268. Daniel, J.M., C.F. Witty and S.P. Rodgers, 'Long-term consequences of estrogens administered in midlife on female cognitive aging'. *Horm Behav*, 2015. **74**: pp. 77–85.

269. Jung, C.G., *Modern man in search of a soul*. 1933, New York, NY: Harcourt, Brace & World.

CHAPTER 10: THE AGEING BRAIN

270. Pew Research Center, 'Growing Old in America: Expectations vs. Reality'. 2009.

271. Jeune, B., JM. Robine, R. Young, B. Desjardins, A. Skytthe and JW. Vaupel, 'Jeanne Calment and her successors. Biographical notes on the longest living humans', in *Supercentenarians*, H. Maier, Editor. 2010, Springer-Verlag Berlin Heidelberg.

272. Buettner, D. '5 Easy Steps to "Blue Zone" Your 2017'. 2017; Available from: https://bluezones.com/2017/01/blue-zone-2017/.

273. Ritchie, K., 'Mental status examination of an exceptional case of longevity J. C. aged 118 years'. *Br J Psychiatry*, 1995. **166**(2): pp. 229–35.

274. Evert, J., et al., 'Morbidity profiles of centenarians: survivors, delayers, and escapers'. *J Gerontol A Biol Sci Med Sci*, 2003. **58**(3): pp. 232–7.

275. Settersten Jr, R.A., 'Relationships in Time and the Life Course: The Significance of Linked Lives'. *Research in Human Development*, 2015. **12**(3–4): pp. 217–23.

276. Mather, M., 'The emotion paradox in the aging brain'. *Annals of the New York Academy of Sciences*, 2012. **1251**(1): pp. 33–49.

277. Belsky, D.W., A. Caspi, et al., 'Impact of early personal – history characteristics on the Pace of Aging: implications for clinical trials of therapies to slow aging and extend healthspan'. *Aging Cell*, 2017. **16**(4): pp. 644–51.

278. Okinawan Centenarian Study, 'Okinawa Centenarian Study'. 2017; Available from: http://www.okicent.org/.

279. NECS. 'Why Study Centenarians? An Overview'. New England Centenarian Study. 2017 [cited 21 October 2017].

280. Perls, T.F. and R. Fretts, 'Why Women Live Longer than Men'. *Sci Am*, 1998.

281. Ostan, R., et al., 'Gender, aging and longevity in humans: an update of an intriguing/neglected scenario paving the way to a gender-specific medicine'. *Clin Sci (Lond)*, 2016. **130**(19): pp. 1711–25.

282.   Camus, M.F., D.J. Clancy and D.K. Dowling, 'Mitochondria, maternal inheritance, and male aging'. *Curr Biol*, 2012. **22**(18): pp. 1717–21.

283.   Sun, F., et al., 'Extended maternal age at birth of last child and women's longevity in the Long Life Family Study'. *Menopause*, 2015. **22**(1): pp. 26–31.

284.   Barclay, Keenan, K., E. Grundy, M. Kolk and M. Myrskyla, 'Reproductive history and post-reproductive mortality: A sibling comparison analysis using Swedish register data'. *Social Science & Medicine*, 2016. **155**: pp. 82–92.

285.   Grundy, E. and O. Kravdal, 'Do short birth intervals have long-term implications for parental health? Results from analyses of complete cohort Norwegian register data'. *J Epidemiol Community Health*, 2014. **68**(10): pp. 958–64.

286.   Boston University Medical Center, 'Reproduction later in life is a marker for longevity in women'. 2014, EurekAlert!

287.   Neu, S.C., et al., 'Apolipoprotein E Genotype and Sex Risk Factors for Alzheimer Disease: A Meta-analysis'. *JAMA Neurol*, 2017. **74**(10): pp. 1178–89.

288.   Alzheimer's Association, '2017 Alzheimer's Disease Facts and Figures'. 2017, *Alzheimers Dement*, pp. 325–73.

289.   Australian Bureau of Statistics, 'Causes of Death, Australia, 2016'. 2017: Canberra.

290.   Prince. M., A. Wimo, M. Guerchet, et al., on behalf of Alzheimer's Disease International (ADI). 'The World Alzheimer Report 2015, The Global Impact of Dementia: An analysis of prevalence, incidence, cost and trends'. 2015, London.

291.   World Health Organization. First WHO ministerial conference on global action against dementia: meeting report. 2015, Switzerland.

292.   Xu, W., et al., 'Meta-analysis of modifiable risk factors for Alzheimer's disease'. *J Neurol Neurosurg Psychiatry*, 2015. **86**(12): pp. 1299–306.

293.   Dementia Australia. 'About Dementia'. 2017 [cited September 2017]; Available from: https://www.dementia.org.au/information/about-dementia.

294.   Irish, M., et al., 'Investigating the enhancing effect of music on autobiographical memory in mild Alzheimer's disease'. *Dement Geriatr Cogn Disord*, 2006. **22**(1): pp. 108–20.

295.   Buckley, R.L. and Y.Y. Lim, 'What causes Alzheimer's disease? What we know, don't know and suspect'. 2017; Available from: https://

theconversation.com/what-causes-alzheimers-disease-what-we-know-dont-know-and-suspect-75847.

296. van Dellen, A., C. Blakemore, R. Deacon, D. York and A.J. Hannan, 'Delaying the onset of Huntington's in mice'. *Nature*, 2000. **404**(6779): pp. 721–2.

297. Fisher, G.G., et al., 'Mental work demands, retirement, and longitudinal trajectories of cognitive functioning'. *J Occup Health Psychol*, 2014. **19**(2): pp. 231–42.

298. Stern, Y., 'Build Your Cognitive Reserve: An Interview with Dr. Yaakov Stern', in *The SharpBrains Guide to Brain Fitness*, A. Fernandez and E. Goldberg, Editors. 2009, San Francisco: Sharp Brains.

299. Vemuri, P., et al., 'Association of lifetime intellectual enrichment with cognitive decline in the older population'. *JAMA Neurol*, 2014. **71**(8): pp. 1017–24.

300. Mattson, M.P., 'Lifelong brain health is a lifelong challenge: from evolutionary principles to empirical evidence'. *Ageing Res Rev*, 2015. **20**: pp. 37–45.

301. Raichlen, D.A. and G. E. Alexander, 'Adaptive Capacity: An Evolutionary Neuroscience Model Linking Exercise, Cognition, and Brain Health'. *TINS*, 2017. **40**(7): pp. 408–21.

302. Ontario Brain Institute, 'The Role of Physical Activity in the Prevention and Management of Alzheimer's Disease – Implications for Ontario'. 2013.

303. Jacka, F.N., et al., 'A randomised controlled trial of dietary improvement for adults with major depression (the "SMILES" trial)'. *BMC Med*, 2017. **15**(1): p. 23.

304. Wahl, D., et al., 'Nutritional strategies to optimise cognitive function in the aging brain'. *Ageing Res Rev*, 2016. **31**: pp. 80–92.

305. Pollan, M., *In defence of food*. 2008, London: Penguin.

306. Johansson, L., et al., 'Common psychosocial stressors in middle-aged women related to longstanding distress and increased risk of Alzheimer's disease: a 38–year longitudinal population study'. *BMJ Open*, 2013. **3**(9): p. e003142.

307. Holt-Lunstad, J., T.B. Smith and J.B. Layton, 'Social relationships and mortality risk: a meta-analytic review'. *PLoS Med*, 2010. **7**(7): p. e1000316.

308. Boyle, P.A., et al., 'Effect of a purpose in life on risk of incident Alzheimer disease and mild cognitive impairment in community-dwelling older persons'. *Arch Gen Psychiatry*, 2010. **67**(3): pp. 304–10.